OUR
DAUGHTERS'
HEALTH

OUR
DAUGHTERS'
HEALTH

Practical and Invaluable Advice for
Raising Confident Girls
Ages 6 to 16

SHARON L. ROAN

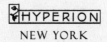

NEW YORK

Library of Congress Cataloging-in-Publication Data
Roan, Sharon L.
    Our daughters' health: practical and invaluable advice for raising confi-
dent girls ages 6 to 16 / by Sharon L. Roan.
        p.   cm.
    ISBN 0-7868-8500-9 (trade paperback)
    1. Girls—Health and hygiene.   2. Parenting.   I. Title.

RA777.25 .R627 2001
613'.04242—dc21   00-038837

Book design by Ruth Lee

FIRST EDITION

4   6   8   10   9   7   5

Dedicated to

KRISTY and JANIE,

two wonderful girls

Acknowledgments

M Y SINCERE THANKS to the people who helped bring this book to life. Foremost, my agent, Julie Castiglia, who was steadfast in her belief in this project and who provided support when I needed it most.

I also wish to thank my editor at Hyperion, Leslie Wells, for her patience and careful work; my husband, Michael Lednovich, for his vast computer-support skills; Susannah Ernst, for her support at the start of this project and for a helping hand near the end; Shelley M. Westmore, Orleda Roa, and everyone at Girls Inc.; Francine E. C. Shannon (Cybermom.com), Kit Bennett (Amazingmoms.com), M. J. Reale (Girlzone.com), and Trish Kasey (MommyTimes.com) for giving me a forum.

I am indebted to *The Los Angeles Times* for granting me time off to write.

Finally, I salute the dozens of families who submitted to interviews and completed my questionnaires. Your concern for your daughters touched and inspired me.

Contents

Preface

Gender differences exist at every stage of human development.
—The Society for the Advancement of
Women's Health Research

As a parent, you've heard all the bad news by now. "Teen girls have high rates of pregnancy." "Smoking soaring among girls." "A quarter of U.S. children are obese." To be sure, there are numerous health threats facing our children—especially our girls. You should be heartened, however, by the vast amount of medical research completed in the past decade showing the many ways we can help our girls become stronger, healthier, less at-risk. This book, for parents of girls ages six to sixteen, will bring that information into your home, into your hands.

Since I became a medical writer in 1982, momentous changes have occurred in women's health. Reporting for newspapers from coast to coast, I have been witness to two decades of "catch up," in which women consumers and activists fought for the same kind of sophisticated medical treatment and research directed at men. It seems hard to believe that, prior to 1990, women were routinely excluded from medical research because of fears that their hormones or possible pregnancies would disrupt clinical trials and because of the blind assumption by doctors that women's bodies functioned similarly to men's.

Today we know that women's health issues are unique and deserve separate consideration. And that is happening. Intense lobbying by the Society for the Advancement of Women's Health Research and the Congressional Caucus for Women's Issues led to a 1993 decision by the Food and Drug Administration to stop excluding women in early-phase clinical trials. This policy change has brought about many new initiatives in women's health, including advances in the diagnosis and treatment of heart disease, breast and ovarian cancer, osteoporosis, and many other conditions that affect women differently than men or in greater numbers. This revolution in medicine has even spawned the largest and most expensive clinical trial ever—Women's Health Initiative—which is expected to yield much valuable information in the coming years. In short, in the last twenty years we have learned a great deal about how women become sick and how they can stay well. But it's time for a second phase of progress. It's time we turn our attention to our girls.

Our daughters are hurting. A look at the statistics in chapter 1 will convince you of that. And research has shown that many of the major diseases and disorders of adulthood have their roots in childhood and adolescence. That girls are accumulating the very same risk factors for poor health that plagued their mothers is tragic and ironic, given the past two decades of progress in disease prevention and health promotion for women.

It's time to renew the commitment to women's health, beginning with our daughters.

A newborn girl today can expect to live eighty years. Whether she will achieve her potential for a lifetime of good health is up to us and what we do for her today and tomorrow. To be sure, it's within our ability to nurture the healthiest-ever generation of women.

SHARON L. ROAN
Orange, California
December 7, 1999

OUR
DAUGHTERS'
HEALTH

CHAPTER 1

Introduction: Raising the Standards for Our Daughters' Health

RECENTLY, I returned to the campus where I attended college after a seventeen-year absence. It was homecoming weekend, and the weather was quintessential Midwestern autumn. I was drawn to the old, cracked sidewalks of the campus and spent several hours walking, enjoying my memories and peering into the faces of the students. Things had changed in my old college town, but it wasn't the sparkling new buildings or high-tech labs that caught my attention. The students had changed. I was struck by how many girls smoked. While some students looked as young and fit as they should be, I noticed that many more young women were overweight. I was told by a college administrator that many students today work one or more jobs to pay their bills, and that time for recreation and exercise was hard to come by. I also learned that the university, like many others, had a severe problem with binge drinking, and that girls' binge drinking rates were closely approaching that of boys'.

In short, the young women looked a whole lot less healthy.

The impression I took home that weekend seemed sadly ironic. Here were girls on the verge of adulthood, pursuing higher education and lofty possibilities in careers, relationships, and life, but who were looking too old for their ages. I don't mean too old in a sophisticated way. I mean too old in that they were showing signs of being saddled with adult health problems: poor nutrition, sedentary lifestyles, substance abuse.

Shouldn't young women seventeen, eighteen, or nineteen years old be at their healthiest?

The answer is yes—of course. But that is not the reality in most girls' lives today. While adult women are demanding top-notch, gender-specific health care, our daughters have one of the worst preventive health profiles of any group. Susan Brenna, the author of a 1999 report in *New York* magazine, summed up the situation on girls this way:[1] "It's counterintuitive that a gener-ation of mothers who are better informed and more watchful of their own health than any before them could be missing the story with their own daughters. Yet a decade's worth of statistics, col-lected by public-health agencies and foundation-funded reports on adolescent health, suggest that girls are in crisis."

Indeed, while we mothers enjoy hard-fought advances in breast cancer, heart disease, and osteoporosis treatment and pre-vention, our daughters are compiling one bad health habit after another that could erode their own chances for vigorous health in adulthood. While mothers are hitting the gym four times a week, our daughters may have long ago stopped playing soccer due to misguided peer opinions about what is feminine or the lack of practice facilities for girls. While we are seeking the best menopausal therapies to stay young and vibrant, some of our daughters may already be at risk for infertility due to the high prevalence of sexually transmitted diseases.

You get the picture. And this picture does not, and should not, cast blame on parents who are doing their best to stay healthy. We should be striving to maintain good health and set an example for our daughters. But it is time we recognize the danger in believing that our daughters are naturally healthy simply because they are young, and that they will remain that way without much attention from us. That may have been the way it was a few decades ago, but it's not that way anymore. Girls today face a different—and far more troublesome—set of health problems than we did. In 1998, the American College of Obstetricians and Gynecologists warned of a generation of young women at increased risk of such problems as depression, infertility, cancer, and osteoporosis unless more is done to support and guide them.[2] To be sure, what we've learned about women's health over the past two decades has a direct bearing on our daughters. We now know that most—not some—major diseases have their roots in childhood.

> "Nearly half of American adolescents are at high or moderate risk for 'seriously damaging their life chances.'"
> —From "Preparing Adolescents for a New Century," the Carnegie Corporation

The Seeds of Poor Health

So why aren't we doing more to put our daughters on the same fast track to good health many adult women are pursuing? There are many factors that have caused both health professionals and parents to overlook girls' health.

It is a popular fallacy that poor health habits in a girl (for

The Risks Facing Our Girls

- Fifty-eight percent of girls say they have been on a diet.[3]
- One in six girls (grades five through twelve) say they have binged and purged.[4]
- One in four children are overweight or obese.[5]
- Twenty-five percent of girls say there was a time when they did not get needed medical care.[6]
- Sixty-six percent of girls have had sex by twelfth grade, and one-third used no contraception the first time they had sex.[7]
- Four in ten teens become pregnant before age twenty.[8]
- One in five U.S. abortions are among teens.[9]
- Eighty-five percent of girls are not getting enough calcium.[10]
- Thirty-four percent of high school girls smoke cigarettes.[11]
- Fifteen percent of high school girls report frequent drinking.[12]
- Eighteen percent of high school girls report using illegal drugs.[13]
- Twenty-two percent of high school girls report they "do not like" or "hate" themselves.[14]
- One in four adolescent girls has symptoms of depression.[15]
- Half of all new HIV cases occur in people under age twenty-five.[16]
- Three million teens are infected with sexually transmitted diseases each year. Half of all cases of chlamydia are among girls ages fifteen to nineteen.[17]
- Twenty-five percent of American children ages ten through sixteen report being assaulted or abused within the previous year.[18]
- Suicide rates among children ages fourteen and younger have increased seventy-five percent in the past decade.[19]
- Forty percent of American children have at least one major risk factor for heart disease.[20]
- Forty-three percent of kids live in households where someone smokes.[21]
- Sixteen percent of children never use sunscreens.[22]
- The ten- to nineteen-year-old age group is the only segment of the U.S. population in which mortality rates have not declined substantially over the past twenty years.[23]

example, a sixteen-year-old who smokes) needn't be of great concern because she is too young to experience much damage, and there is plenty of time for her to get back on track. But what is particularly dismaying about risky behaviors that begin in girl-hood is that habits, values, and lifestyles established during this period are likely to continue throughout life. And statistics sug-gest that many girls are already heading down the wrong road.

Like many parents, you may be misled into thinking that girls are easier to protect from harm than boys. To be sure, boys are not as healthy as they used to be, either, with higher-than-ever rates of obesity, substance abuse, and HIV. Many boys suffer men-tal health consequences from living in a society that imposes a narrow and constrained version of masculine behavior. And boys may be more vulnerable to health risks such as sports injuries or automobile accidents.

But girls are "catching up" to boys in certain risky behaviors, such as substance abuse. Girls suffer far more from such silent health risks as disordered eating and depression. Girls are far more likely to be victims of abuse and harassment than boys. Girls still receive far fewer opportunities at sports and recreation than boys. Moreover, girls' unique biology means that they suffer greater consequences from such problems as sexually transmitted dis-eases, sedentary lifestyles, and air pollution.

"The fact is, girls experience adolescence differently than boys do. While both boys and girls engage in risky behaviors, we know that young adolescent girls are less likely to engage in physical activity. More likely to have a negative body image. More likely to be depressed. And more likely to attempt suicide."

—Dr. Vicki Seltzer, American College of Obstetricians and Gynecologists

Self-Rated Health Status

Girls realize that their health is not as good as it could be. Boys, however, do not seem to experience the same decline in health during youth that girls do.

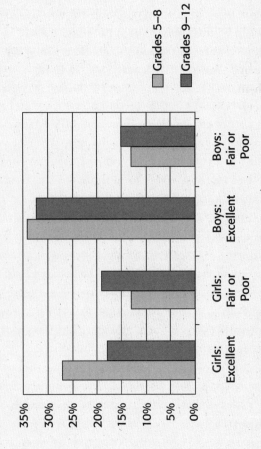

Source: Commonwealth Fund.

What Is Happening to Our Girls?

Unhealthy habits in girls tend to accrue quietly and insidiously, and parents are not noticing. It's not surprising that our daughters' accumulation of subtle but serious risk factors for disease slip by us. Surely, there is nothing as lovely as a growing girl. And it's natural to think of all children in the age range of six to sixteen as healthy. It's particularly easy to be complacent after the high-maintenance years of baby and toddler-hood and put health concerns aside. A survey by *Prevention* found that eighty-five percent of parents are mistaken in the belief that their children are in good or excellent health. Good health is not just the absence of disease. It is a lifestyle that honors and protects the body and preserves its functions.

Perhaps you may not fully realize the potential risks facing your daughter. A 1998 study of middle-school students found that parents and students agreed that certain things such as not wearing seat belts and using diet pills were risky. The parents who were surveyed tended to recognize obvious health risks, like dieting, but downplayed the consequences of dieting compared to how their daughters perceived the threat. It's interesting that the girls themselves understood better how harmful this behavior was compared to their parents. As parents, we are too often in the dark about issues that our children see as serious risks, such as the prevalence of weapons at school, and drug use.

Perhaps we need to consider how much the world has changed since we were young—changes that undermine our efforts to raise healthy children. Our changing environment is one factor (violence and pollution are more serious threats, for example). And cultural influences, such as our penchant for restaurants and fast food and heavy use of computers and TV, may contribute to the erosion of good health. There is also evidence that society's efforts to "equate" the sexes and offer a full range of

Parents typically fail to understand how many issues are a threat to their children's health. This survey asked middle-school students and their parents how prevalent certain risky behaviors were.

	Students		Parents	
	Yes	No	Yes	No
Weapon in school	25%	75%	2%	98%
LSD, cocaine use	7%	93%	0%	100%
Suicide attempt	22%	78%	2%	98%
Has sex	58%	42%	2%	98%
Alcohol use	55%	45%	5%	95%
Tobacco use	48%	52%	14%	86%
Marijuana use	62%	38%	3%	97%

Source: Thomas L. Young, M.D., and Rick Zimmerman, Ph.D., *Archives of Pediatric and Adolescent Medicine*, Vol. 152. November 1998. The survey was of 194 middle-school students and their parents.

opportunities to women has led us to drop a layer of protection around our girls. In the book *The Body Project*, Cornell researcher Joan Jacobs Brumberg argues that the turn-of-the-century environment has become the enemy of girls. Not only do girls mature physically earlier than ever, they are faced with fewer social protections. This situation "leaves them unsupported in their development and extremely vulnerable to the excesses of popular culture and pressure from peer groups," Brumberg writes.

On one hand, feminism has helped us create overdue freedoms for girls, such as the 1972 Title IX legislation that ended discrimination on the basis of sex and opened up more sports opportunities to girls. We try to teach our girls to be confident, assertive, and to demand their rights. We want our daughters to be strong, independent, autonomous, and responsible—all important aims. But there is a potential downside if we turn our girls loose without the skills and resources to guard their own interests. Brumberg points out that close female relatives, usually the mother, used to be the people to teach girls about their bodies and health. Today, the role of teaching girls about physical, mental, and sexual maturity too often falls to ill-prepared schools, too-busy doctors, television, advertisers, or uneducated peers. The early maturation of girls' bodies coupled with the bombardment of negative female images in the media is a recipe for disaster for too many girls.

> "In my judgment, no group is more at risk than are young girls. They're growing up in a culture that's being carpet-bombed each day with the message that not only are you never too young to have sex appeal, you're also never too young to worry about it."
> —Donna Shalala, Secretary of Health and
> Human Services

To be sure, it's harder today for us to shield our daughters from the big, bad world. Materialism, violence, the threat of AIDS, raw media images, and the decline of good role models all throw new challenges before parents. Family life has changed, too, and it is often strained. By 1990, more than half of all mothers of young children and school-aged children worked, and there is little evidence that with more mothers working, fathers are making more time for their kids.[25] According to one survey, U.S. children today have ten to twelve hours less of parental time compared with kids in the 1960s.[26] Close to half of all kids live through divorce by the time they reach sixteen. And only about 5 percent of children see a grandparent regularly.

> "Many of the current statistics are, indeed, discouraging. But such findings should compel concerned adults to redouble their efforts

to enable girls to envision and strive for optimum health for both mind and body."

—From the National Council for Research on Women, "The Girls Report: What We Know and Need to Know About Growing Up Female," 1998.

As parents become busier and more harried, children are expected to take on more responsibilities, some of which may be too much too soon. In particular, most girls need support and advice on how to cope with pressure from peers to engage in behaviors that may be risky. You need to rethink the trend of pushing your daughter too quickly into the adult world. She may very well appreciate your taking some of the pressure off her to fend for herself or make decisions that she's not ready to make. What girls really want is your closeness and protection. Instead of giving girls freedoms to venture into dangerous corners of the world or freedoms to set their own values, we need to aim for giving them a more valuable type of independence—one that emerges from close and loving relationships with their parents and that stems from girls' own confidence in themselves and their abilities and talents.

Girls Gaining Ground

There are bright signs, however, that adults—parents, doctors, public health officials, researchers, and policy makers—are waking up to the health risks confronting our daughters. In 1996, the Department of Health and Human Services under Secretary Donna Shalala, launched a nationwide campaign to encourage and empower girls to adopt healthy behaviors, beliefs, and habits. The campaign is based on the idea that girls possess naturally proactive attitudes about their health when they are eight or nine and that we can reinforce and sustain these values for the long term. The good news for you and your daughter is that campaigns like Girl Power have begun to focus on what we can do to keep girls healthy—and there is so much we can do. There have been no less than three dozen reports (either governmental, foundation-sponsored, or academic) on various aspects of girls' health in the 1990s and countless other studies and projects. These analyses

---

What Does It Mean to Be a Healthy Girl?

Not a great deal is known about robust health in childhood. In the report "The Future of Children," Dr. Barbara Starfield of Johns Hopkins University writes: "Although much is known about the health problems of children and adolescents, little is known about their health." She goes on to explain what is becoming so apparent to experts in women's health: "The absence of a medically defined disorder does not prevent individuals from feeling ill or from being at risk of an abnormally short life span."

People tend to think that children and adolescents are healthier than others because they have fewer medically definable illnesses. But often, illnesses are simply at an earlier stage in children and teens, Starfield says.

So what is health? Is it just a clean report from the doctor at an annual checkup? The World Health Organization defines children's health as "a state of complete physical, mental, and social well-being and not merely the absence of disease or infirmity."

A healthy girl, then, is a "complete girl—her social, physical, emotional, and cultural environment—rather than just one aspect of a girl's experience."

Sources: "The Future of Children," report of the David and Lucile Packard Foundation, Winter 1992; World Health Organization; The President's Council on Physical Fitness and Sports; and The Center for Research on Girls & Women in Sports report "Physical Activity and Sport in the Lives of Girls," April 1997.

What Do Adolescent Girls Need for Healthy Development?

Parents and other family members can:

- Serve as positive role models by showing respect for girls and women, and expressing confidence in girls' aspirations.
- Embrace all aspects of girls' identities—including their sexuality, their perspectives, and their priorities—and provide a respectful context where girls can raise questions and voice their concerns.
- Encourage girls to do well in school by discussing their studies with them, exploring potential areas of interest, supporting their achievements, and becoming involved with girls' schools.
- Encourage girls to explore their strengths and develop their talents in all fields, especially those not traditionally thought of as "female."
- Advocate for equal programs, facilities, equipment, and publicity for girls and boys in school- and community-based athletic programs, and support the involvement of girls who have traditionally not seen themselves as athletes.
- Help girls to respect their bodies and discourage the development of eating disorders by rebutting negative cultural messages about body image and encouraging healthy behaviors.
- Provide access to nonjudgmental information and resources to prevent unwanted pregnancies and the transmission of HIV/AIDS and other STDs. Offer guidance and support to help girls make decisions about a range of types of sexual activity.
- From a young age, foster girls' sense of entitlement to respectful treatment and to teach them that they can speak out against behaviors of others that hurt them.
- Support girls' involvement in community groups and extracurricular activities, help them to develop leadership skills, and encourage them to take action to promote constructive social change.
- Raise boys in ways that foster their respect for girls and women.

Source: National Council for Research on Women, "The Girls Report: What We Know and Need to Know about Growing Up Female," 1998.

have cited other positive trends. Girls today are more bold, determined, smart, and resilient.[27] They recognize the odds stacked against them and are willing to be partners for change.

There are also signs that some negative health trends have already hit bottom and are improving. Girls are doing better in reading and math. The teen birth rate has fallen, and more girls are using contraceptives. A recent surge in drug use has leveled off. Several new magazines for girls have been created that focus on normal-sized girls instead of waifish models. More girls than ever are participating in sports.

With your support, your daughter can ride the crest of these positive trends and create a new standard for what is healthy during the youth and adolescent years. But parental involvement is key.

Parents: Promoters of Healthy Habits

You play a significant role in creating a healthy environment and instilling values and information that will give your daughter the best chance of vigorous, lifelong health. That doesn't simply mean making sure that she eats nutritiously or is encouraged to exercise. It also means teaching her how to express her opinions, stand up to peer pressure, and recognize the cultural forces that portray women differently from how we really are.

This book is a call to action. As parents, we cannot depend on schools to help us raise healthy girls. The Carnegie Corporation report on adolescents called health and life curriculum "the weakest link in middle grade school reform."[28] And at the 1997 meeting of the American Psychological Association, researchers presented several studies showing that various very popular "prevention" programs for kid—such as Drug Abuse Resistance Education, or D.A.R.E., school-based sex education programs, and the Children's Television Act—have all largely failed to meet their prevention goals.[29] Finally, our health care system has sometimes let down girls, particularly in adolescence, as we shall see in the final chapter of this book.

As parents, you already know intuitively that it's a big mistake to let your daughters learn about their bodies, sexuality, nutrition, and other health issues from their peers. Adolescent behavior is largely shaped by peers and by the media. You need to compete with those influences and act aggressively to counter misinformation. For example, research has shown that kids typically overestimate the number of their peers who are doing risky things. One easy and effective thing you can do is to tell your daughter that not everyone is doing what she suspects.

> "My parents and I talk about everything—drinking, drugs, feelings. My friends and I talk about everything, too, but sometimes I can't believe what they say. My parents tell me stuff so I don't have any misconceptions."
>
> —Stephanie, age fifteen

Families, it seems, matter greatly in children's adoption of healthy habits—probably more than you think. One study of almost 1,500 high school students found that students who placed a high value on good health, understood the consequence of risky health behavior, and had parents who modeled good health habits indeed exhibited better health habits.[30] The researchers also found that feeling good about school, having friends who participated in conventional activities like youth groups and community volunteer work, involvement in safe social activities, and church attendance correlated with good health habits.

Your daughter wants and needs your firm guidance well into her late teen years. A landmark 1997 survey of 12,000 adolescents, grades seven through twelve, found that families are more important at discouraging children from taking major health risks than previously suspected.[31] "There's been a pretty significant myth that peer groups are important and parents are not," said Dr. Robert Blum, one of the researchers who worked on the National Longitudinal Study on Adolescent Health. "We've focused so tremendously on peer pressure and instituted so many things to deal with peer pressure. And what this study is saying is that family environment matters most." The survey showed that teens who said they were close to their families were least likely to engage in risky behaviors, such as drug use, smoking, and having sex. Children tended to have healthy habits if their parents had high expectations for their school performance and tended to be home at key times during the day (such as after school, dinner, and bedtime).

In particular, parental expectations for their children's bright futures are crucial. The survey also found a strong protective factor in parents who consistently express feelings of warmth, love, and caring to their kids. This doesn't necessarily mean spending large amounts of time with your daughter. Being home at certain times, for example, wasn't found to be as important as emotional closeness. "What this study showed is that it is emotional availability, far more than physical presence, that makes the difference. You need to give your kids the message that when they need to talk to you, you're available, even if it's by phone, and that they matter," the authors of the study concluded.

You also need to reinforce good health habits by "walking the walk." Research has concluded that teens closely model their parents' health habits regarding smoking, eating, and exercise.[32] Even more impressive was the finding that teens will not pick and choose which of their parents' habits to model and instead tend to mimic their overall "health-risk lifestyle." Thus, if the parents had several poor health habits, the teen would tend to emulate all those habits as well. Conversely, extremely healthy parents tended to have extremely health-conscious teens. Boys tended to follow their fathers' examples while girls' repeated their mothers' habits.

Talk ... and Listen

As your daughter moves into the adolescent years, you can look for opportunities to support healthy behavior in your con-

---

Kids need to know they can trust and count on their parents, according to these findings from the KidsPeace survey of ten- to thirteen-year-olds.

- Seven out of ten kids feel that when they need help they can count on their parents to be there and do what's best for them.
- Seventy-one percent said they are more comfortable speaking to their mothers than their fathers.
- Only four out of every ten kids say they feel their parents always spend a lot of time with them.
- Seventy percent of preteens feel their parents don't always understand what it's like to be a kid.
- Kids feel their parents usually offer helpful advice. Six of ten say when they have spoken to their parents about serious problems and concerns, their parents were very helpful. One-third said their parents were somewhat helpful.
- One-third of the kids feel that sometimes their parents still treat them like little kids. Two-thirds said they feel treated like a person their age should be treated.
- Sixty-seven percent say their parents always treat them with respect.

Source: 1995 National Preteen Survey: "A Report to Congress and the Nation," KidsPeace, The National Center for Kids in Crisis.

versations with her. Perhaps the single most important tactical step you can take to ensure that your daughter will enter adulthood healthy is to learn how to talk and listen to her meaningfully. This might occur because she asked you a question (such as, why do so many of her friends diet?). Or perhaps a situation arose while you were watching television with her (for example, a character decides to attend a rave party). These are the so-called teachable moments, when you find your daughter is interested and receptive to hearing what you have to say.

Talking to your daughter about health could easily turn into discussions about the risks she faces—and your fears. But reciting statistics and revealing your anxieties won't influence your daughter in a positive way. Scaring her with statistics won't help her feel good about herself or in control of her future well-being. Instead, encourage your daughter to respect her body, avoid dangers, and develop beliefs and practices that will sustain her emotionally and physically.

Indeed, for the most part, it is she who will arrive at the decision to practice good health habits because of the examples you set and the way you support her as she arrives at her decisions.

> "The relationship I have with my mother is very different than the one I have with my father. In order to stay close to my mother, we go shopping. She always lets me skip one day of school a year to go shopping for an entire day. We go out to lunch, just the two of us, and have a whole lot of fun together. In order to stay close to my father, we play board games, throw around the softball, or go fishing. He is the parent who helps me with my homework. And I ask him for advice on guys, because he was one once."
>
> —Cheka, age fifteen

It may seem hard to communicate, especially with a teenager. But experts have come up with many good tips. For instance, be aware of when your daughter seems receptive to talking (sometimes it's in the car or late at night). Don't ruin the opportunity by lecturing. Deliver information in droplets and then let your daughter comment or ask questions.

A window of opportunity exists between the ages of ten and twelve.[33] During these years, parents are kids' primary source of information, guidance, and advice. But as kids reach the teen years, they turn more to other sources of information. You shouldn't hesitate to take on hard topics, even when your daughter seems too young to handle such matters or hasn't inquired much about a particular issue. It's natural for you to feel a little inept. But these discussions are too important to avoid having. Moreover, it's a wonderful opportunity not just to dispense infor-

Parents are not giving their children enough information, according to a 1999 Kaiser Family Foundation survey of 880 parents and 346 kids.

Percentage of parents and kids who say:

	Kids ages 10–12 want more information on topic	Parents of kids 10–12 who never talked about it
How to protect against HIV	50%	40%
How to handle pressure to have sex	44%	46%
How to know when you're ready to have sex	43%	50%
How to prevent pregnancy/STDs	38%	62%
What kinds of birth control available	32%	68%

Source: Kaiser Family Foundation/Children Now, "Talking with Kids about Tough Issues," 1999.

mation but to make your values and expectations clear to your daughter.

"You have a real feeling that you want to protect your child and keep your child as innocent as you can for as long as you can. While that's a laudable goal, your kids are being exposed to information," notes Matt James, president of the Kaiser Family Foundation, a nonprofit national health care philanthropy based in Menlo Park, California.[34] You may be reluctant to bring up topics because you fear your daughter will inquire about your own past. Perhaps that's why surveys show that conversations on sex are the most difficult for parents, with one in five kids saying their parents were unprepared for a talk. "It may be one of those things where you're preaching, 'Do as I say, not as I did,' " says James. "I think that's hard for parents. Many of us who grew up in the sixties, seventies, and eighties probably engaged in premarital sexual activity. What you say to your kids may be different than what you actually did." James advises that kids "will take as an answer: 'We're not going to get into what I did when I was young. But this is what Mom and I think is right for you.' It's not dodging something. Kids will accept these boundaries."

Tips for Parents from "Talking with Kids about Tough Issues"

1. Create an open environment. Kids will turn to parents for answers only if they sense that parents are receptive to their questions. Don't give negative responses to questions just because they are hard, you are not in a good mood, or it's an inconvenient time. It's okay to buy some time, but express your interest in answering it and then follow through.

2. Consider your child's temperament. Answers should be tailored to whether a child is a worrier or outgoing, etc.

3. Respect your child's feelings. If children can express their feelings, it increases the chances they will come to you with problems and questions.

4. Understand the question. Don't give a young child more answer than she is looking for. If you're unsure of what a child is asking, ask the child some questions first to get an idea of where she's at.

5. Always be honest. Your child will trust you to tell the truth. If you don't give a straightforward answer, kids will make up their own fantasy explanations.

6. If you don't know something, admit it. Kids will accept that you don't know everything and will appreciate honesty.

7. Don't leave big gaps. You don't have to tell a child all the details, but don't leave major facts covered up or children will make up their own answers for those knowledge gaps.

8. Use age-appropriate language. It can be tempting to fall back on medical terminology, but kids may not understand big words. Think about what your daughter is likely to understand.

9. Get feedback. After having a discussion, check back with your child to see what she remembers and understands.

10. Be patient. Let kids tell you the full story. Listen patiently and let the child speak at her own pace. You'll find out more and you'll let your child know that she is worthy of your time.

11. Say it again and again. You can't have one big talk. Give children bits and pieces over time on a particular topic. They'll keep asking questions; sometimes the same ones. Repetition helps them learn and understand.

12. Give them your undivided attention. Stop what you're doing and sit down with your child. Make eye contact. It adds conviction to your message and helps build your daughter's self-esteem to let her know she is worthy of your full attention.

13. Speak separately to kids of different ages. If children are not very close together in age, speak to them separately to tailor the discussion to each child's developmental stage.

14.   Other tips from the Kaiser booklet "Talking with Kids about Tough Issues": Start early; communicate your own values; use TV as an educational tool.

Source: Kaiser Family Foundation and Children Now, 1999.

Youth: The Springboard to a Healthy Life

You won't raise a girl who is in perfect health. That's impossible. Some good habits will stick; some won't. Some children will be receptive to parents' efforts; others will be very difficult to reach. Personalities, disabilities, circumstances, environments, culture, ethnicity, and economics all figure into the mix. Parents need not be perfect and need not be the perfect role model. But we can educate ourselves about good health and demonstrate to our daughters our sincere efforts to take care of ourselves. We can demand more attention for our girls from our health care providers. We can make a strong case to our daughters for adopting good health habits. We can teach our girls to respect their bodies. We can protect them from risks. We can promote the ideal that our daughters have the right and expectation to enter adulthood at the peak of good health: physically, mentally, and emotionally.

CHAPTER 2

Strong Bones:
A Window of Opportunity

I T   W A S   a beautiful spring day in Southern California. At a regal Beverly Hills hotel, 500 women had dressed in their finest luncheon dresses to attend a women's health conference. A panel of some of the nation's top experts in women's health were seated at a table on the stage. They spoke of how women could protect themselves from breast cancer, heart disease, and other ailments.

"But what about osteoporosis?" asked one woman, rising from her seat in the audience. Clearly, osteoporosis, which affects mostly females in the later part of life, was of importance to these women, many of whom envisioned themselves still playing tennis at eighty. Who wanted to be hunched over or in a wheelchair or having hip replacement surgery instead of being mobile and active at eighty? Osteoporosis, a degenerative disease that affects 25 million Americans, is the cause of many of the broken bones and fractures that plague elderly women.

A doctor on the panel, one of the nation's leading authorities on the disease, patiently described to the women that they should exercise and could take hormone therapy to help prevent bone loss.

"What about calcium?" the woman demanded. "Will it help?"

Yes, said the doctor, adding a caveat: It can help maintain the bones but will not add mass to the bones. That process ends when a woman is about twenty-one. Indeed, the doctor added rather bluntly, "If you really want to prevent osteoporosis, drink a lot of milk when you're twelve."

A collective groan rose among the women. And yet, no doubt many of them went home, eyed their daughters, and went to work to prevent them from having to worry about osteoporosis someday.

Osteoporosis is a "pediatric disease with geriatric consequences," says Dr. Duane Alexander of the National Institute of Child Health and Human Development.

Osteoporosis Prevention in Childhood

Four factors appear to be extremely important in the development of osteoporosis. They are calcium intake, exercise, hormones, and heredity. You can do a lot about the first two factors; not much about the second two.

The female hormone estrogen plays a key role in bone health. After menopause, when estrogen production declines, women start to lose large amounts of bone mass. Thus, the presence of estrogen appears to be important in protecting bone. There is also some evidence that girls who begin to menstruate later than average (thirteen and older) have lower bone mineral density, perhaps because they have gone longer without exposure to high levels of estrogen.[1] If your daughter meets this description, you should be cognizant of the special need for adequate calcium intake.

Heredity also figures strongly into the development of osteoporosis. Osteoporosis and bone fractures occur in higher rates in ethnic and racial groups. Moreover, some families with a history of osteoporosis may have genetic defects that prevent optimal calcium absorption.[2] In particular, some people carry genes that slightly impair the function of vitamin D, which is crucial to bone growth.[3] This can lead to a higher risk for osteoporosis. It's not certain, however, if increased calcium consumption can offset the genetic tendency toward osteoporosis. For these families, the prudent advice is to consume at least the Recommended Daily Allowance (RDA) for calcium.

It's also clear that Caucasian women of Northern European ancestry and Asian women have a higher rate of bone fractures. African-American girls, however, appear to absorb calcium more efficiently and form new bone at a faster rate than whites. Women of Mediterranean descent also seem to have lower rates of osteoporosis. But ethnic groups with lower rates of osteoporosis are not immune from the disease, and these girls should make sure they are getting the RDA for calcium despite their lower risk for bone problems.

Another risk factor is being thin. This is the reason why: The more body fat a woman has, the more estrogen she produces. And estrogen appears to help slow the rate of bone loss. Smoking is another risk factor because smoking decreases estrogen in the body. There is also some evidence that smoking interferes with calcium absorption and the bone-building process.

Calcium Matters Now

This chapter is entitled "A Window of Opportunity" because you can make a big difference in your daughter's bone health no matter what your heredity. It is imperative that all girls get plenty of calcium in their diets up through about age twenty. Dietary calcium is the mortar of bones. The more consumed, the more that is available to increase bone mass up to a certain point. (Beyond this maximum point, further calcium intake won't contribute to skeletal mass.) The body's ability to build bone ceases at about twenty or twenty-one. After that time, the body can recycle or lose calcium but cannot add it to bones. The higher an individual's bone mass at its peak in early adulthood, the lower the risk of osteoporosis. In other words, it's now or never for your daughter to build bone. Forty-five percent of her peak bone mass will be formed during the years of birth to age ten.[4] Ninety percent of the peak mass is formed by age seventeen. What this means is that a girl who hates milk and doesn't consume other calcium-rich foods could end up with fully 10 percent less bone by early adulthood compared to a girl who consumes enough calcium.[5]

But how much calcium does your daughter need?

In 1997, the National Academy of Sciences, a non-profit organization, issued new recommendations to increase childhood consumption of calcium.[6] The academy put the optimal values as follows:

- Children ages 1 to 3: 500 mg daily
- Children ages 4 to 8: 800 mg daily
- Children ages 9 to 18: 1,300 mg daily

Fahra, whose daughter Callie is seven, has watched her calcium consumption closely since age two. "I think it's extremely important that my daughter get enough calcium in her diet. I think the earlier we start stressing this, the better." If your child is meeting the RDAs for calcium, that's terrific. Be aware, however, that some experts suggest that the threshold level—the optimum amount of calcium that contributes to bone strength—should be even higher than the current Recommended Daily Allowances for children and teens; up to 1,500 mg a day for adolescents. But most children and teenagers get nowhere near enough calcium. More than eight out of ten teenage girls don't meet the RDA for calcium.[7] Most girls consume about 797 mg of calcium a day, only 66 percent of their RDA.[8]

> "Researchers would love to have young girls eat a good diet and maintain good bone status throughout their lives, as part of a plan to reduce the risk of suffering a hip or spine fracture later in life. An added advantage of this would be that society wouldn't have to bear the attendant cost of treating these maladies. But that's not happening. Given the way things are going currently, these girls are a public health catastrophe waiting to happen."
>
> —Gordon Wardlaw, Ohio State University
> researcher

Calcium matters greatly throughout childhood. But growth spurts should serve to remind you that that growth has to be supported by something. Studies have shown high bone-forming activity in girls as young as five. And the years just before and after puberty appear very important.[9]

Putting Calcium into the Diet

Some girls are likely to have even more trouble than most getting enough calcium. Athletes are one such group. While your daughter may be consuming her RDA in calcium, that amount may not be enough if she is highly active. Activity increases the body's need for nutrients, including calcium. Studies show the spines of some young female athletes are as weak as women in their seventies and eighties.[10] This does not mean that exercise is bad for girls' bones. On the contrary, physical activity combined with an optimum calcium intake appears highly protective of bones.

Camp Calcium

One summer a few years ago at Purdue University, fourteen girls ages twelve to fourteen attended an unusual kind of summer camp. It was called Camp Calcium. The camp consisted of a three-week summer vacation at a sorority house and was, by all accounts, tons of fun. But the girls had a job to do as well: They had to eat the same food, including snacks; give blood and collect all their body wastes for researchers who would monitor every nutrient that came in and went out of their bodies. The girls had to drink all of their milk and eat every bite of yogurt and ice cream served to them. (Their diet contained about 1,332 mg of calcium, similar to the RDA.) They had to rinse out their cartons of milk with deionized water and then drink the water. But the researchers put their young subjects' efforts to good use. At the end of the study, the scientists were able to show that these girls—during a key time of life for skeletal development—*put about five times more* calcium to use for their bones compared to a group of women ages nineteen to thirty-two who followed the same protocol. The young girls retained about 326 mg of calcium a day out of the 1,332 mg they consumed. The young women ages nineteen to thirty-two retained only 73 mg per day.[12]

While it may sound like the girls lost a lot of the calcium they took in, never underestimate the value of that extra glass of milk per day—you know, the one your daughter surreptitiously pours down the sink before dashing off to get dressed for school. An extra serving of a calcium product each day, such as a slice of cheese or extra glass of milk, can accumulate over your daughter's youth to dramatically boost her bone density. A modest increase of about 350 mg of calcium a day—about one glass of milk—could greatly boost bone density in twelve- to fourteen-year-old girls.[13]

"Young girls not yet in high school may be setting themselves up for osteoporosis—simply because they are not consuming enough calcium-rich foods. It's absolutely critical for these girls to achieve optimum bone density to help make bones less susceptible to fractures and breaks both now and later in life."

—Dr. Gary Chan, professor of pediatrics at the
University of Utah

Chronic dieting also is a risk factor for osteoporosis because it can lead to a decreased consumption of milk and other dairy products. Some girls may think high-calcium foods, such as milk, are fattening and avoid them due to concerns about losing weight or lowering their fat intake.[11] But your daughter can get adequate amounts of calcium without adding to body weight.

The Importance of Physical Activity

You and your daughter should look at calcium intake during the ages of five to twenty as similar to putting money in the bank. Ask your daughter to picture how she wants to look at seventy. Julie's mother is sixty-eight and already has such severe osteoporosis that she is beginning to suffer a curvature of her spine. She has discussed Grandma's problem with Marcia, fourteen. "I really worry about Marcia getting enough calcium. She doesn't seem to care too much. I point out the problems that her grandma has because of a lack of milk when she was a kid."

Encourage your daughter to participate in physical activities in addition to getting enough calcium. Physical activity is crucial for girls for many reasons (which we will explore in several other chapters). Strong bones is one reason. Generally, it's suggested that physical activity may explain about 6 to 20 percent of variation in bone mineral measurement. Bone, like muscle, is a living tissue that gets stronger in response to exercise.[14] It adapts to the level of stress placed on it by forming more tissue—or losing it. Activity seems to help increase a woman's bone density until about age twenty-one. Bone size, but not density, can increase until about age twenty-six. All kinds of exercises, such as running, basketball, even nonweight-bearing exercise like swimming and biking, are effective in increasing bone density. One study found that athletic participation in high school increased the mineral content of the hip bone by about 7 percent.[15]

But a high activity level doesn't mean that girls can skimp on calcium.

Milk and Other Sources of Calcium

"I think it's so important that Erin get calcium in her diet, but she does not like milk and I have a hard time trying to make sure she gets the calcium she needs," says Rita, whose daughter is nine. "I have her take a Tums antacid to help her get enough."

Let's face it, it's not easy to get children and teens to eat large amounts of calcium-rich foods, especially if they don't like milk. Remain observant of your daughters' diets, even in those busy-busy teen years. If you leave it up to your daughter to get enough calcium, she probably won't. Teens often think they are getting far more calcium than they are. One poll of girls ages eleven to fourteen found that most claimed they were drinking at least one glass of milk per day.[16] But data show that almost half of all teens don't drink any milk at all.

Kids may think that they have "outgrown" the need for milk, but dairy foods are, plain and simple, the best source of calcium. Milk, yogurt, cheese, and other dairy products account for about 75 percent of Americans' calcium intake. If your daughter doesn't eat dairy products, it's very hard to get enough calcium. Experts call milk "a nearly perfect food" that includes vitamin D, which is necessary for the body to absorb calcium and create bone mineralization.[17] Young adults should also get 200 IU of vitamin D (which can be found in dairy products, cod liver oil, fatty fish, and is created in the body by exposure to sunlight).

Milk also has vitamin A, which helps vision, cell growth, and the immune system; protein, which maintains and repairs muscles; potassium to regulate fluid balance in the body; riboflavin for converting food into energy; niacin, which helps enzymes function in the body and metabolizes sugars and fatty acids; phosphorus, which builds strong bones and generates energy from food, and vitamin B-12, which builds red blood cells.

You shouldn't succumb to your kids' complaints about milk. The anti-milk attitude of teens is something unique to recent generations. Milk consumption has declined over the past three decades. Kids also skimp on calcium by skipping meals, eating snack foods, and eating foods away from home (especially fast-food restaurants—how often does your child want a Coke instead of milk with her Happy Meal? Hint: Insist on milk. No milk, no fast food). Besides the increase in skeletal mass, adolescents need lots of calcium because they may have poorer absorption rates of the nutrient. The current RDA for calcium assumes that 40 percent of the calcium teens take in is absorbed. But teens may actually absorb only 26 to 35 percent of their calcium intake.[18]

Teens should consume 1,200 to 1,500 mg of calcium per day, which is about four or five servings of dairy products. Some calcium-rich foods include:

One and a half ounces of mozzarella cheese, 269 mg
Eight ounces of milk (whole, 2%, 1%, skim, organic), 315 mg
Eight ounces of soy milk, 80 mg
One cup plain yogurt, 292 mg
One cup cooked collards, 350 mg
Half-cup almonds, 200 mg
One cup canned baked beans, 163 mg
Half a can salmon, with bones, 242 mg

Teens' fondness for salty foods increases urinary calcium excretion and plays a role in this low absorption. The more sodium a person eats, the more calcium is excreted in the urine.[19] For example, a teen girl eating 10,000 mg of sodium a day in potato chips and fast food could be losing close to 300 mg of calcium.

Soft drinks, too, appear to have out-muscled milk on kids' menus. Two-thirds of girls drink 23 ounces of soft drinks a day.[20] One in four teens has soft drinks with dinner.[21] In fact, high cola intake itself is associated with an increased risk of bone fractures in girls. Excess protein in the diet can also cause an increased purge of calcium in the urine. Too much protein is, in general, a problem in the typical American diet.

How to Look for Calcium on Food Labels

Calcium is one of only four vitamins and minerals that must be listed on food labels. You can always find it. This label, for a macaroni and cheese product, shows that one serving provides 15 percent of the recommended amount of calcium needed each day.

Kids who have lactose intolerance should still be able to get enough calcium in

Nutrition Facts

Serving Size 1 cup (228g)
Servings Per Container 2

Amount Per Serving

Calories 260   Calories from Fat 120

	% Daily Value*
Total Fat 13g	**20%**
Saturated Fat 5g	**25%**
Cholesterol 30mg	**10%**
Sodium 660mg	**28%**
Total Carbohydrate 31g	**10%**
Dietary Fiber 0g	**0%**
Sugars 5g	
Protein 5g	

Vitamin A 4%	•	Vitamin C 2%
Calcium 15%	•	Iron 4%

* Percent Daily Values are based on a 2,000 calorie diet. Your daily values may be higher or lower depending on your calorie needs:

	Calories:	2,000	2,500
Total Fat	Less than	65g	80g
Sat Fat	Less than	20g	25g
Cholesterol	Less than	300mg	300mg
Sodium	Less than	2,400mg	2,400mg
Total Carbohydrate		300g	375g
Dietary Fiber		25g	30g

Calories per gram:
Fat 9 • Carbohydrate 4 • Protein 4

Tips for Getting Kids to Like Calcium:

- Pizza is a good choice; don't forget taco pizza, veggie pizza, and barbecue pizza. A slice of cheese pizza has 220 mg of calcium. Veggie pizza is a healthy choice and has about 300 mg of calcium.
- Try kid favorites like cheese enchiladas, tuna and shells with cheddar sauce. A half-cup cheddar cheese in a dish adds 150 mg of calcium.
- Think about calcium snacks such as string cheese (one serving contains about 300 mg of calcium), fruit-filled yogurt (300 mg).
- If your daughter dislikes white milk, try chocolate. A spoonful of chocolate syrup added to an 80-calorie cup of skim milk may do the trick without adding fat.
- Add milk to soups, rice, scrambled eggs, and oatmeal. Three tablespoons of nonfat dry milk can be added to baked goods, or meatloaf and increases the calcium value by about 160 mg.
- Smoothies with mixed fruit, ice, and milk make a good snack and provide about 315 mg of calcium if a full cup is used.
- A great source of calcium is orange juice fortified with the nutrient; it provides about 300 mg of calcium. Look for the specially labeled orange juice cartons.
- Breads and cereals also have extra calcium added. Kellogg's Nutri-Grain Cereal Bars are good sources of calcium (400 mg per bar). Cereals fortified with calcium contain about 150 mg per serving.

reduced–lactose milk, which can be found in most grocery stores. If your child refuses milk, or if your child or your family practices a strict vegetarian diet, it will be essential to include other high-calcium foods into your daily diet, such as sardines (153 mg per serving), salmon (242 mg), tofu (130 mg), and broccoli (38 mg). Other foods high in calcium include kale (47 mg), turnip greens (99 mg), kidney beans (90 mg), and sesame seeds (100 mg). Look for foods fortified with calcium, such as orange juice and some grain products. "Kellie drank plenty of milk for most of her life," says mother Bridgit. "But last year she had a stomach bug and threw up some milk. She then associated milk with her illness and has refused to drink it. So I discovered orange juice with calcium, and she loves that." Betty has stressed to her two daughters that some vegetables contain both calcium and other nutrients: "I have talked to them about the media campaign to make people think milk is the only source of calcium when, in fact, many vegetables are a good source."

The key is to make calcium consumption easy, available, and enjoyable. Ask teens what "deposits" they have made in their bone bank each day. They'll think you're corny, but you'll be keeping calcium in the conversation. Point out that healthy hair, skin, and teeth reflect a diet with plenty of calcium. The insides benefit, too; you just can't see it. Remind kids of what is at stake here: How many bones about it? Two hundred and six! And they are mostly made up of calcium.

What about Calcium Supplements?

Should you give your daughter a calcium supplement? Certainly, most adult women rely on supplements to get the calcium they need to maintain bones. Supplements intended for adults are widely available. Calcium supplements intended for children are usually found in children's multivitamins. For example, Flintstones has a multi that comes with extra calcium. However, that vitamin contains a modest 200 mg of calcium, or one-sixth of what girls need daily.

There is little research on how effective calcium supplementation is for growing girls. One study showed that teens who added 700 mg per day of calcium to their diets improved their bone mass by 10 percent. But when 300 mg to 700 mg of calcium supplements were added, teens bone mineral increased only between 1 and 5 percent. Dairy products may be more effective in depositing calcium because of the composition of other nutrients in the food. Moreover, supplements shouldn't be taken indis-criminately. Excess calcium intake is associated with the development of kidney stones in susceptible people.

Questions to Ask Your Doctor

- Would my daughter benefit from undergoing a nutrition evaluation with a nutritionist?
- I'm told that medicines like anti-inflammatory drugs for arthritis and asthma, anticonvulsants, and thyroid supplements can cause bone loss. My child is taking a medication that can prevent calcium absorption. Is there a way to offset this, or should I give her additional calcium?
- My daughter has had two fractures and one broken bone in separate incidents. Should she undergo a bone density test?
- How much will a vegetarian diet prevent my daughter from getting enough calcium?
- Should my daughter take a calcium supplement? Which one?

Resources

- For more information about high-calcium diets, call the National Dairy Council: 800-426-8271. A jazzy brochure for girls on the importance of calcium can be obtained. It's called "Power Up From the Inside Out."
- For more information on osteoporosis, call the National Osteoporosis Foundation: 202-223-2226.
- "Clueless About Calcium" is a booklet from the National Institute of Child Health and Human Development and other organizations that help girls understand the importance of calcium. Call 800-WHY-MILK.
- Teens can visit the Clueless in the Mall web site to participate in a fun game that will educate them on calcium. Visit www.calcium.tamu.edu.

CHAPTER 3

Skin Care: Act Now, Rejoice Later

Margaret and her daughter, Seana, eight, live within a stone's throw of the ocean in Florida. Not surprisingly, they are at the beach "almost every weekend," says Margaret. But mother and daughter are not typical beachgoers. Margaret keeps a firm eye on her wristwatch and every half hour calls Seana over for another liberal helping of SPF 15 sunscreen. "She sometimes gets a little pink on her cheeks. But she has never had a sunburn in her life," Margaret says, proudly.

Seana sometimes complains about the sunscreen interruptions. But someday, she *will* thank her mother. Never underestimate the importance of skin care among women. Think about it. How many of us wish we hadn't worked so hard for that suntanned face of our youth? How many of us wish we had responded faster to our first serious case of acne? The skin is the largest organ of the body. It acts as a shield to protect the body against disease, infection, and the environment. It is part of our appearance and thus helps define who we are. Nice skin tells the world that a girl is healthy. You need to be watchful of two major problems that can seriously impact your daughter's skin (and, perhaps, her self-esteem) for the remainder of her life: Sun exposure and acne.

Tanning Is Definitely Uncool

Kids love the sun. Heck, we all love the sun. But the sun is bad news to children, especially fair-skinned ones. Eighty percent of an individual's lifetime exposure occurs during childhood.[1] Early sun exposure, especially tanning and sunburns, causes the vast majority of the skin cancers and sun-damaged skin that occurs during adulthood. Even one or two severe sunburns during childhood dramatically increases the risk of developing skin cancer as an adult, including the dangerous and often-fatal disease melanoma.[2] "Skin cancer is one of the few diseases that can be minimized if people protect themselves from the sun," says Dr. Lynn Drake, president of the American Academy of Dermatology.

As parents, we can no longer ignore piles of medical research demonstrating the clear dangers of even moderate sun exposure. And studies show that how parents approach sun protection will strongly influence their children's lifetime sun protection habits. Pam, whose daughter is thirteen, has made protection from the sun a health habit for her family. "I am always concerned about sun exposure," she says. "I always make sure my daughter is wearing sunscreen in the summer when she's outside for more than half an hour. I don't promote tanning."

Using sunscreens is perhaps the most important habit to adopt because children spend a lot of time outside. Outdoor activity is usually great for kids. But less than half of all children use sunscreens.[3] And sunscreen alone is often not enough or is not used correctly.[4] Many children suffer sunburns even after putting on a sunscreen of SPF 15 or higher. Why? Kids typically don't put on enough (a full ounce, or about a palmful is needed to cover most exposed skin) and don't reapply sunscreen every two hours or after sweating heavily or playing in water. Sunbathing greatly increases the risk of burning. Discourage this old-fashioned practice, which will only give your daughter more wrinkles later in life.

Girls are also less likely than boys to wear a hat outdoors. Point out to your daughter that boys wear baseball caps and that girls can, and should, wear head protection, too. Connie, who lived for a time in New Zealand, learned much from the way that country has addressed epidemic skin cancer rates. "My daughter always uses sunscreen when out in the sun for long periods of time. The kids in New Zealand are taught at school about the dangers of sunburn. Most of our schools will not allow the kids to go outside at lunchtime if they are not wearing a hat. The message is pushed on TV and in magazine advertisements."

There are a number of ways to protect children from sun damage.

- Avoid going outside during the hottest part of the day, especially the hours between 10 A.M. and 4 P.M.
- Cover bare skin that burns easily. For example, don't hesitate to wear a T-shirt over a bathing suit. When you're out of the water, drape a towel over your exposed skin. Wear a hat. Use UVA/UVB-blocking sunglasses to protect your eyes. Several manufacturers now make bathing suits for children and adults that are designed

to cover more skin and block out harmful rays. Many swim shops carry this clothing during the summer months.

- Don't forget to use sunscreen on winter days when the sun is still bright (for example, while skiing) or on warm but cloudy days.
- Use a sunscreen with an SPF of at least 15 with both UVA and UVB protection. If you have fair skin, use an SPF 30 or higher.
- Apply sunscreen thirty minutes before you go out. Put more on after swimming or sweating heavily.
- When applying sunscreen, use enough to fill your palm. Don't be stingy.
- Use "waterproof" sunscreen if you are going into the water.
- Avoid surfaces like water or snow that can reflect the sun's rays.

Sunscreens work by absorbing, reflecting, or scattering the sun's rays on the skin. There are many types, and you should have no trouble finding one your child likes. Some of the newer forms include stick sunscreens that make application to the face easier, spray sunscreens, and suncreen "towelette" wipes that make application to the body simple and thorough. If your daughter resists using sunscreen, look around for a product marketed for girls, such as ones that go on colored (such as in pink or purple). Younger kids, like Linzey, thirteen, seem to be learning that the sun can be harmful. "I don't sit in lawn chairs all day drowning myself in tanning spray stuff," says Linzey. "I have fun! I won't go outside without sunscreen. My bro didn't wear sunscreen and his back is peeling like the leaves off a tree in the fall." Take advantage of this kind of attitude and help your child adopt a habit of skin protection.

Caution your daughter against using indoor tanning parlors. According to health experts, fifteen to thirty minutes in a tanning salon is equivalent to an entire day at the beach.[5] Ultraviolet A radiation from tanning beds may even be related to the most serious form of skin cancer, melanoma. Tanning beds can weaken the immune system and cause dry skin and burns.

Know Your Skin Type

Skin type	Sun history	Examples
I	Always burns easily, never tans, extremely sun-sensitive skin	Redhead, freckles Irish, Scots, Welsh
II	Always burns easily, tans minimally, very sun-sensitive skin	Fair-skinned, fair-haired, blue-eyed, Caucasians
III	Sometimes burns, tans gradually to light brown, sun-sensitive skin	Average skin
IV	Burns minimally, always tans to moderate brown, minimally sun sensitive	Mediterranean-type Caucasians
V	Rarely burns, tans well, sun-insensitive skin	Middle Eastern, some Hispanics, some African Americans
VI	Never burns, deeply pigmented skin, sun-insensitive skin	African Americans

Source: Food and Drug Administration.

Acne

"I hate zits," says Karly, thirteen. "You have horrible bumps on your face, and no one will ever have a crush on you. I can't make them go away."

It is a painful paradox for adolescents. Never before have there been so many effective and quick treatments to prevent and treat acne. But society's attitude about acne hasn't changed. Too many people still believe that acne is an acceptable part of adolescence. That all kids get it. That it's no big deal. But acne is a big deal. A bad, or even relatively mild, outbreak can cause a self-assured girl to lose her confidence, drop out of activities, and begin to think of herself as a loser. "Acne caused me deep-rooted despair," says Suzanne, whose problems with acne began at age thirteen. "It's like having a terminal illness. It almost destroyed me."

> "Acne is an assault on a teen's self-image and affects what they will do—whether they will try out for the school play, athletic teams, or class office. It makes them more reticent, less outgoing, less willing to take a chance. It really has a negative effect on their ability to relate to people."
>
> —Dr. Diane Baker, dermatologist

Teenagers with serious acne feel embarrassed and anxious. And, a survey by the American Academy of Dermatology showed that girls are more likely than boys to say that acne made them self-conscious and made them like themselves less. Many girls lack self-esteem due to their complexion or worry that the acne affects the way people react to them when meeting them for the first time. Astonishingly, surveys find only 16 percent of teens with acne see a doctor and only 13 percent use prescription medications, which are often far more effective than over-the-counter acne products.[6] "I think the psychological effects of acne are underestimated," said the study's author, Dr. Diane Baker, a Portland, Oregon, dermatologist.[7] "Even for kids with cases that are not severe, it is embarrassing to them, and their self-esteem suffers at a time when self-esteem is already fragile. But for years, it's been the impression on the part of parents of teens that this is something that you have to put up with."

Carrie has seen how acne has changed the way her daughter thinks about herself and even acts. Her daughter Rachel, now thirteen, began breaking out at eleven. "My daughter is semidevastated by her acne. She sees girls who do not work as hard as she does at school, who are quite self-centered and rude at times but who have gorgeous complexions. Her acne is not the worst case I've seen but it's not as simple as a small, occasional pimple. She refuses to wear a bathing suit in front of others because of the condition on her back. She has been struggling with this for two years and it's beginning to take a toll on her emotionally."

Acne Myths and Realities

- Sweating leads to facial acne breakouts. *Reality: There is no direct correlation between sweat and acne.*
- Moisturizing clogs the pores, leading to acne. *Reality: Although heavy cream-based products are not good for maintaining clear skin, it is always important to moisturize the skin, even while experiencing breakouts. Be sure to stick to noncomedogenic products.*
- Drinking a lot of water will clear up a bad complexion. *Reality: While hydration is important for overall skin health, it will not prevent acne.*
- Scrubbing the face will clear up acne. *Reality: It is important to always treat the skin gently. Wash your face with a mild cleanser no more than twice a day.*
- Eating greasy foods causes acne. *Reality: Foods do not cause breakouts, regardless of the amount of grease or oil they contain.*
- Ignoring acne will make it go away. *Reality: Leaving skin untreated will not clear a bad complexion—it will only exacerbate the problem.*
- All acne medications are the same. *Reality: Visiting your dermatologist is the best way to determine which products are the best for your skin type.*
- Acne is caused by stress: *Reality: Stress is a factor in aggravating acne but does not cause it.*

Source: Ortho Pharmaceutical News.

Acne occurs in 80 percent of girls during adolescence.[8] It often begins earlier and lasts longer than in boys, but boys tend to have more severe cases. Five percent of all teens will have such severe acne that permanent scars are left.[9] Even milder forms of acne can leave scars. Acne is largely triggered by rising hormone levels that cause the oil glands in skin to get bigger—not by stress, chocolate, or even dirt or poor hygiene. Teens tend to blame themselves. "There is a guilt about it," says Baker. "They think, 'It's my fault that I have this, and I have to suffer with it.' "

You can do a lot to help your daughter avoid the misery of acne. First, if you have a family history of acne, particularly the severe, cystic acne, take your daughter to the doctor as soon as signs of acne begin. It's even wise to consult a doctor if your daughter has a mild or initial case of acne because it's impossible to tell how bad the acne might become. Make it your goal to prevent severe acne instead of waiting until it has become a horror for your daughter and then reacting. Mild cases of acne can be helped by some over-the-counter products containing benzoyl peroxide. It often takes four to six weeks for these products to work.[10] But if any treatment isn't working by six weeks, you may need to try something else.

Prescription antibiotics or Retin-A, a cream, usually work well with mild or moderate acne. It is imperative, however, that your daughter use highly protective sunscreen on her face when using Retin-A. The active chemical in the medication causes sun sensitivity. Severe sunburns can occur without ample use of sunscreen. More severe cases of acne may need treatment with the drug Accutane, which works very well but is a real danger if your daughter should become pregnant while taking it. Accutane taken during pregnancy is associated with a high risk of severe birth defects. Thus, if your teen is prescribed Accutane, a doctor may also ask that she take oral contraceptives as well—even if she is not sexually active. Oral contraceptives, incidentally, can often have a positive effect on acne.

You can also help by being sensitive to how much acne embarrasses and distresses kids. When acne first becomes a problem, it's easy for parents to say nothing and act like they haven't even noticed. They may feel that acknowledging the acne will make the child feel even worse. But that is not the case. Ask your daughter if her acne is bothering her, and explain that it can be successfully treated. Remind your child that it will clear up and that acne doesn't change who she is and all the things about her that are beautiful. "If I don't at least take it seriously and let her know that I feel her pain, she might feel more alone than an emerging adolescent girl already does," notes Pamela, whose daughter is fourteen and has serious acne. "It would be insensitive and unloving not to help her and just think that this is a passing phase. She needs to know that someone cares and doesn't minimize the importance to her. She needs to hear from others that she won't be scarred for life."

And that emotional support includes doctors. Helen has been unhappy about the clinical, remote manner of her daughter's dermatologist and is currently looking for a pediatric dermatologist. "Although this doctor is a competent, nice guy, he is not invested in his patient's age the way he needs to be. My daughter is not just a case of acne but is a growing, thriving young girl."

Piercing

Angela has two holes in each earlobe, a ring in her naval, and a gold stud in her nostril. Angela, if you haven't already guessed, is pretty darn normal. Piercing is the current generation of teenagers' unified statement of independence and identity.

While many girls will settle for a few holes in their ears, many more will want additional piercings. "I think pierced ears look really neat," says Julie, eleven. "I want one more hole at the top of my ear and another in the earlobe!"

How you decide to handle the piercing phenomenon is a personal matter. Some families tolerate it, while others think it's inappropriate behavior. But health experts do have some good advice if you decide to ride the piercing wave. Serious complications from piercings are rare.[11] Very infrequently, piercing can cause HIV and hepatitis from dirty needles. The bigger problem is in the wide range of mild to moderate health problems related to piercing that aren't rare at all. These include skin infections, scarring, broken teeth from biting down on a tongue stud, and speech impediments from a tongue stud.

To prevent problems, have piercing done by someone who is trained and who meets the standards set by the Association of Professional Piercers. In general, piercing guns should be avoided and only instruments that are taken out of sterile bags just prior to piercing should be used. Think hard about whether the risks of tongue and nose piercings are worth it. Besides the problems already mentioned with tongue piercing, some teenagers have aspirated the tongue stud, and wounds can become contaminated with bacteria and food. The nose is sensitive because the cartilage can be mistakenly pierced instead of the soft tissue. That can lead to scar tissue that causes the nostril to be pulled up. Problems can occur in the ears, too, if cartilage is pierced instead of soft tissue. Any time an area that is pierced becomes red, itchy, or irritated, see a doctor.

Any piercing should be followed up by rigorous after-care. Any doctor or good piercer will give your daughter instructions for how to clean and care for the wound for several weeks.

Nickel Allergies

DeeDee, fifteen, remembers the ugliness like it was yesterday. A friend had pierced her ears with a sewing needle and an apple. Within a few months, her ears itched, a large, raised red bump appeared next to the openings, and an itchy rash spread on her neck below her ears. "It was so gross," she says.

Nickel allergies are an all-too-common consequence of body piercing among girls. Nickel in inexpensive jewelry is the fastest-growing and biggest cause of contact skin rashes in America.[12] Nickel allergies have increased a whopping 40 percent in five years.[13] About 10 percent of all females have nickel allergies.[14] Because girls often can't afford to buy 14-karat gold earrings and opt for inexpensive jewelry, they are prime targets to develop a nickel allergy. Nickel allergies are more common in the summer when sweat leaches nickel from metal.

There are ways to avoid nickel allergies. First, have your daughter's piercing done by a pro. Demand that she use surgical stainless-steel or gold earrings for the first year. You can also buy a nickel test kit and check jewelry using a cotton swab. There is also nickel-safe jewelry on the market, such as Simply Whispers (see Resources).

Other Skin Concerns

Moles

Moles are very common and can range widely in shape, size, and color. Most appear during childhood. Many moles will become darker and larger during the teen years. New ones may even appear. Certain types of moles have a higher than average risk of becoming cancerous. Consult your pediatrician about any moles your child has. Sometimes doctors will recommend that certain moles be removed prior to adulthood to reduce the risk of the skin cancer melanoma.

Cold Sores

Cold sores or fever blisters are caused by the herpes simplex virus. This virus typically runs in families. It can cause blisters and sores almost anywhere on the skin but most frequently on the mouth, lips, and nose. The chin and cheeks can also be affected. It is transmitted by kissing or using the same drinking glasses or towels. Once a child has a herpes outbreak, the virus stays in the body and sores can recur. Excessive sun exposure, illness, and fatigue can bring on an outbreak. If the problem becomes serious, resulting in frequent outbreaks, consult a dermatologist. There are several new oral medications that can dramatically curb outbreaks, and these medications are safe for children.

Eczema

Eczema can occur in childhood. In fact, some children are scolded for scratching when parents don't realize that they actually have eczema. If your child scratches excessively, see a doctor. There are good medications to treat the disorder.

Dry Skin

Dry skin is very often hereditary. So if one or both parents has it, watch for it in your daughter. Light-skinned people tend to be more prone to dry skin. Use lotions liberally and see a doctor if skin becomes so irritated that it bleeds or cracks.

Warts

Warts are caused by the human papilloma virus. Often, parents deem warts not serious and wait for them to go away on its own. While that certainly may happen, a competing scenario is that warts will spread, even to other parts of the body. The best advice is not to wait. Take your child to the dermatologist with the first wart and have it treated.

Don't hesistate to call a dermatologist if you are concerned about a skin problem. While primary care doctors can often diagnose and treat minor skin ailments, dermatologists have the expert training to know when a condition warrants specialized treatment. Dermatologists treat people of all ages. Some dermatologists specialize in treatment of children and teens.

Questions to Ask Your Doctor

- What is the best sunscreen for my particular child (taking into consideration her skin type, amount of time spent in water, region where you live)?
- Are all sunscreens safe for children?
- Is my child's acne mild enough to be treated with over-the-counter products or do we need prescription treatment?
- Can you reassure my child that the acne will clear up? Can you give us a time frame for about how long it will take to see her complexion improving? Is there anything she can use now to safely cover up the acne?
- What kind of soap should my daughter use on her face?
- Can you refer me to a doctor who does piercing or a piercing parlor that follows stringent safety practices?
- My daughter gets frequent cold sores. Can you give us a prescription medication to have on hand so that we can treat it at the first sign of an outbreak?
- Are my child's moles unusual or a potential problem later in her life? Should they be removed, and at what age?

Resources

- Source: American Academy of Dermatology; www.aad.org or call 888-462-DERM.
- Simply Whispers nickel-free jewelry; 800-451-5700 or visit Hypoallergenic.com.
- Information on skin protection is available from the American Cancer Society at 800-ACS-2345 or at www.cancer.org.
- The Ortho Dermatological company, which makes products to treat acne, has a web site for teens that explains the condition and how kids can cope. Visit www.pimpleportal.com.

CHAPTER 4

Body Image and Self-esteem:
How Your Daughter
Pictures Herself

"Being yourself, in actuality, is fairly difficult. Media messages tell us to be a certain shape and size, our friends and peers want us to like certain things, our parents wish we'd act a specific way. With all the different messages from all different angles, it is sometimes hard for a girl just to find the person she really is."

—Gabriella, age fifteen

WHEN THE EDITORS OF *Seventeen* magazine decided to add a fashion spread to their January 1998 issue featuring adolescents who wore larger sizes, the response couldn't have been more striking. The feature, showing girls wearing trendy outfits in sizes 14 and 16, garnered nationwide attention and praise. The feature was prompted in part by letters and E-mails from readers who wanted more of the magazine's content to focus on real girls who come in all shapes and sizes. The feature led to other articles about helping girls embrace their uniqueness. One article pointed out that clothing manufacturers are becoming interested in larger-size, cool clothes for girls and discussed how larger-size girls shouldn't adhere to fashion "rules" that plus-size women traditionally succumb to—such as wearing solids, long sleeves, and big skirts. Indeed, the *Seventeen* spread showed its models in trendy camisoles and long, narrow skirts. Eventually, several magazines for girls focusing on physical diversity were launched.

The *Seventeen* article, and the reaction to it, are positive signs that women are trying, to some extent, to free girls from the confining cultural ideals of beauty that have compromised women for decades. Despite these promising signs that our culture is redefining beauty for our daughters, we have a very long way to go. The reality is that a girl growing up today has a far better chance of falling into the old, mentally and physically harmful belief systems concerning beauty than she has in embracing a healthier alternative. The media—particularly magazines, television, and movies—are a major reason why our girls erroneously learn from a very young age that they must look a certain way in order to be successful, happy, popular, and content. We mothers, too, sometimes inadvertently reinforce this defeating philosophy in our daughters. As many as 75 percent of American women perceive themselves as overweight, and up to 80 percent diet.

Indeed, to foster healthy self-images in our daughters, we need to examine ourselves and our culture. In a laudable television special, actress Rosie O'Donnell and journalist Linda Ellerbee addressed the body-image problem. During the show, kids discussed where their feelings about body image come from, what the media's role and responsibility is in shaping this fantasy, and how to identify the difference between a poor body image and who they really are.

> "Kids, more than ever, are mistaking looks for personal worth and happiness. Dieting is beginning earlier and earlier and the average age for anorexia in young girls is now eight. This special will not only give them a chance to speak freely about their looks, but will, hopefully, inspire them to change the world and how it judges people, because our generation has failed miserably."
>
> —Linda Ellerbee, Nick News Special Edition,
> "The Body Trap"

Dieting isn't the only consequence of growing up obsessed about physical appearance. Some girls go to great lengths to change their appearance. The number of girls under age eighteen who are undergoing cosmetic surgery doubled from 1992 to 1996—their parents obviously buying in to their daughters' pleas that only a drastic physical change will make them content.[1] Other girls who lack confidence in themselves due to physical imperfections tend to look for affirmation from others—especially boys. From this shaky platform, girls may be easily persuaded into actions and behaviors that are not in their best interests. These girls will do almost anything in order to be sought-after and admired.[2] Carey, fourteen, has dieted herself into a serious eating disorder: "I was once very, very heavy; when I was around eight until the time I was fourteen. In fact, I started making myself throw up in second grade to get away from the mean chubby jokes I got. To me, being thin is everything. *Everything*."

Multiplication Tables . . . and Dieting

How did we create a society in which girls as young as nine or ten are worried about their body image? The popular media has a lot to do with it. Over the last half of the twentieth century, a beauty esthetic favoring thinness has evolved in the United States. The media has been instrumental in helping create a beauty standard that is nearly impossible to attain. This image—of the tall, slender, large-breasted, flawless-skinned woman—is presented as typical or prevalent. A study looking at girls' attitudes of body image found this vision of the ideal female body is widely accepted among girls.[3] The teenagers in the study described the perfect girl as 5 feet 7 inches, weighing just over 100 pounds, with long legs and long hair. "The ideal girl was a living manifestation of the Barbie doll," the researchers concluded. The consequence of nurturing this hallucination is that those girls who don't turn out to look this way—the majority—may be left feeling like failures; people who will never measure up in what appears to be the most important of attributes. Says Marguerita, fifteen: "I'm always wondering what people are going to think of me. Are they going to like the way I dress? If somebody says something mean about how I look, I feel so bad."

Poor body image has numerous grave consequences for our daughters. Poor body image is a significant factor in the development of depression in some teen girls. There appears to be a specific time in a girl's development, usually the pre-adolescent years, when she begins to doubt herself on all levels.[4] A girl's feelings about her uniqueness and even her goals for herself become eroded by her realization that society may have already defined a narrow role for her: one that emphasizes how she looks and devalues her opinions. It's no wonder that this realization can lead to depression and desperate measures to re-seize control, such as by dieting and adopting destructive health behaviors.

"I wanted to be on the swim team this year," says Adrianna, fourteen, a high school freshman. "But then I thought, how am I going to be in a bathing suit? I don't have a nice body. I decided, okay, I'm going to get in this sport; I'm going to lose weight over the summer. The summer came and nothing happened. I couldn't get in shape because I was used to eating a lot. I decided to forget it. I really wanted to be on the swim team, but I'm afraid people will say 'you're too fat.' "

Often, the first manifestation of a girl's loss of self-confidence is a fear that her body does not match society's stereotypical ideal. So common is girls' dissatisfaction with their bodies that dieting has become something of a wayward developmental step in childhood.[5] Some girls as young as eight expect to be dissatisfied with their bodies and begin to diet as if it is an inescapable part of growing up; a kind of "rite of passage," says one research psychologist.[6] Don't mistake dieting as a positive sign. It might seem like a sixth-grade girl who is dieting is exercising control, maturity, and social awareness. Dieting may make a girl feel that she's fitting into her peer group, since dieting is so common a behavior. But it has many negative consequences.

A study carried out by the National Heart, Lung and Blood Institute looked at 2,379 girls ages nine and ten and drew some surprising conclusions:

- Forty percent of the girls had tried to lose weight (a group that included girls who were normal weight or underweight).
- The girls most likely to try to drop weight were those who were overweight or those whose mothers had told them they are heavy.
- The girls who were dieting actually consumed only slightly fewer calories than those who weren't.

You should address the roots of body dissatisfaction before your daughter reaches age eight or third grade. Sometime during the pre-puberty years, around fourth through sixth grade, girls' thoughts about their bodies shift. This change in attitude precedes, sometimes by several years, a girl's actual attempts to diet or alter her appearance.

Your Daughter Is Watching You

While culture is one powerful influence on girls, adult women, especially mothers, are another major influence. Girls observe their mothers and model themselves after them, particularly at young and impressionable ages. If your daughter hears you complaining about your weight, obsessing in front of the mirror, and talking about another diet, you can be sure that she will consider whether she, too, should be worried about her body and her weight. There is a strong relationship between mothers and daughters in both eating patterns and mood states. That is, if you diet and are depressed about your body, chances are your daughter will adopt the same pairing: dieting and depression.

If you grew up worried about your weight, avoid deflecting this worry onto your daughter. If your daughter is overweight or even chubby, it's natural for you to want her to be thinner. But a healthy weight should never come at the expense of her precious body image and view of herself as competent, normal, and cherished. One study found that one in three girls was on a diet, and half of those dieting were doing so with their mother's encouragement.[7]

Your daughter needs more calories than you and is likely to put on weight during puberty. This is normal and shouldn't be cause for alarm—or a diet. Andrea asks her daughter, Mia, fourteen, to be patient while her body grows and evolves during puberty. "She worries that she is fat. I try to explain that her body is changing rapidly." Another approach is to sit down with your daughter and a family photo album and point out the range of body shapes and sizes in the family. Praise this diversity.

"Save your daughters the pain of what you went through."
—Rebecca Manley, the Massachusetts Eating
Disorders Foundation

Racial Differences in Body Image

Fortunately, not all girls are susceptible to dissatisfaction with body size. While white girls often aim for an unattainable ideal body, black girls typically express other characteristics as being more important to self-image, such as style and personality. In one study, more than 70 percent of the African-American girls expressed satisfaction with their current weight. These girls possessed a more "flexible" ideal that was not cast in a particular size or image and emphasized a sense of personal style and flair. Another compelling finding of this study concerned how girls view one another. The white girls tended to be envious of girls who were closest to the image of the ideal girl, while the African-American girls described themselves as being more supportive of one another and receiving positive feedback from family members, friends, and community members about "looking good." Shanniece, fifteen, described her satisfaction with her body this way: "I know I look good. I don't like anyone telling me how to do my look. My look is my own." This attribute should be praised and protected in African-American families. But parents should be aware that as more opportunities become available in society for women of color, adhering to a cultural ideal of the perfect body might become an issue for black girls, too.

What accounts for these racial differences? There is little research on this question. Some experts have suggested that black girls may benefit from having strong female role models within their families. In other cultures, families clearly place a premium on males. Consider what familial, ethnic, or cultural beliefs have been transmitted through your own families and how you might break or replace those negative traditions in time to spare your daughter. Vanna, the mother of Miki, eleven, is determined to help her daughter think differently about body weight. "There is a good possibility that she will tend to gain weight easily, and I want this to be something she can handle with a good attitude so that it's not a worry or constant problem for her. She has seen her father, older brother, and me worry about our weight and we are all currently working on eating better and getting away from dieting. When other girls are around we discuss things like body types and accepting what you can't change. So far I think we've succeeded in keeping the focus off weight and more on developing her inner self and working on developing the gifts she has."

The Connection Between Poor Body Image and Risky Health Behaviors

It's natural to worry if your daughter is heavy or eats too much junk food. It's tempting to step in and help your child control her weight. Surely, you don't want to see your daughter subjected to the teasing and discrimination that often accompanies weight problems. And, it's true that being overweight in childhood poses numerous serious health risks. You may feel as if you're caught in an impossible position of wanting your daughter to attain an optimal weight for good health and yet not wanting to contribute to obsessive attitudes about body shape and size.

A full discussion of this troubling paradox is contained in the chapter on weight. For now, let's briefly consider the current advice most health experts give to parents. These dictates are: A) feed your child a balanced, healthy, nonrestrictive diet; B) encourage regular physical activity; and C) promote the belief that if you do A and B, whatever shape your body takes is the one you're meant to have, and should take immense pride and pleasure in. How to obtain that delicate equation will be discussed more fully in the chapter on weight.

The reasons for promoting a healthy self-image as your primary goal are many. While it is true that being terribly overweight can trigger many health consequences, feeling awful about

This study showed that girls who dieted tended to succumb to other risky health behaviors (17,135 girls surveyed).

	Girls who never dieted	Girls who always dieted
Binge eating	15.4%	43.4%
Fear can't stop eating	5.6%	35.9%
Tobacco use (weekly or daily)	16.4%	23.3%
Alcohol use (weekly or daily)	13.4%	22.1%
Cumulative drug use (greater than 2 drugs)	49.8%	68.4%
Suicide risk (high)	13.1%	21.0%
Sick days (greater than one day)	39.7%	49.8%
Sexual intercourse (ever)	29.7%	41.6%
Physical abuse (ever)	10.7%	18.8%
Sexual abuse (ever)	12.7%	19.6%

Source: Simone A. French, et al., *American Journal of Public Health*, May 1995, Vol. 85. No. 5, pp. 695–701.

your body is equally, if not more, devastating to a developing girl. Dieting itself, according to many studies, seems to be a gateway behavior to other self-defeating behaviors.[8] Weekly or daily alcohol or tobacco use is about one-and-a-half times more prevalent in girls who always diet compared with those who never diet. Suicide risk, sexual intercourse, and physical or sexual abuse increase in prevalence with frequent dieting. Dieting is also correlated with poorer family relationships and family stress.

The development of eating disorders may be another consequence of dieting at very young ages. Girls who diet tend to binge more often.[9] Girls who purge are half as likely to have a positive body image and three times as likely to have a history of binge eating.

Offering Our Girls a Different View of Themselves

You can counter the destructive voices that might cause your daughter to question her very self-worth. One of the most powerful ways is to help your daughter become a critical observer of media images of women. The media helps shape kids' perceptions of themselves and the world. Your daughter receives much of her information about society and culture through the filter of the television screen. Thus, to influence her beliefs about body image, you need to start by becoming a vigilant media watchdog.

It should come as no surprise to parents that television and other forms of media can be a poor influence on children and adolescents. The average child spends twenty-two hours a week watching TV.[10] Violence, disrespect, and sexual behavior are pervasive. One study found up to eight sexual messages per hour of programming during the so-called family hour. Children's TV shows have the smallest percentage of female characters, and most of the female characters are only interested in boys and clothes.

Most female images in fashion magazines also come off as completely one-dimensional. This fact is not lost on Barbara, thirteen. "When you look at people in magazines, there are so many things about them that you want to be like. Some girls I know starve themselves to be skinny like the models. They try to change their whole way of being. I worry about how I dress, how I wear my hair."

The more girls dwell on thin female stereotypes on TV, in movies, and in magazines, the higher their risk of developing an eating disorder.[11] This saturation of sexual material in the media is particularly harmful to girls because it is combined with increasingly relaxed cultural attitudes about sex and less protective attitudes on the part of parents over what their children see, hear, and know.

Harping at what your daughter is watching on TV won't help. In fact, sometimes our girls think we are criticizing them when we make negative remarks about kids' television shows, books, toys, games, etc. Be careful to point out that you object to the forces in the media that are directing harmful content at your daughter. Sometimes, humor is a useful tool to point out sexist media material. You can wonder aloud why it is that a woman would wear high heels to a picnic, for instance. Play a game with your daughter: Count how many household product commercials feature a woman performing domestic tasks compared to a man.

It's not hard to find examples of sexism. An annual event known as the Good, the Bad, and the Ugly Awards is held each year by a group of women in advertising to bring attention to the pervasive use of sex in sales pitches for products. The group is highly effective at pointing out sexist and demeaning ads against women while promoting ads that empower and praise women. One recent Ugly award went to a taco company that promoted an item called a Macho Combo Burrito and featured a bikini-clad woman running in slow motion. Girls are invited to comment and judge the commercials, and as eleven-year-old judge Sara Smith noted: "What does a woman in a bikini have to do with tacos?" That is exactly the kind of comment you can make to your daughter should the commercial air when you are watching television together. Point out examples of female degradation, sexism, and misogyny. Your daughter will soon develop her own eye for it—and her own indignation.

Efforts have been made to reduce the amount of violence on children's television and to limit gender bias and sexual exploitation. But don't fool yourself that a television-ratings system and some nominal efforts are really making a difference. Entertainment and the marketing of products are the primary reasons that television exists. Even television news is subject to ratings wars and sensationalism that sometimes focuses on the worst in mankind. Girls, in particular, seem to be affected by the news, whether it's on television or in the newspaper.[12]

There are many good books, brochures, and programs to help you teach your daughter about media literacy. Several are listed in the Resources section. Here are some other tips from the Los Angeles–based Center for Media Literacy:

1. We are active when we watch TV. How we interpret TV has to do with our life experiences. But we can filter and change what TV presents by the way we watch it. We can teach our kids that we can challenge, question, and contradict what we see and hear. Talk back to the TV in front of your children. If you don't say anything, they'll assume what they're seeing and hearing must be okay with you.

2. TV's world is made up. Everything in media is constructed by talented photographers, writers, editors, artists, actors, musicians, and others. Their goal is to keep viewers interested and involved. Discuss how they do this.

3. TV makers use identifiable techniques. We can take apart the world that the media constructs by identifying camera angles, music, special effects, and things that make a scene scary or alluring. Kids do not always realize how they are being manipulated by the power of these techniques. Count the laugh tracks in a sitcom or the number of times the music changes in a show in order to demystify TV.

   Another way to identify how the media constructs a world that's not completely "real" is to ask certain questions of the media. The next two tips suggest important questions we can ask:

4. TV teaches us that some people and ideas are more important than others. All media carry subtle messages about who and what is important. There are victims, heroes, and heroines. Some characters are glamorized and others are treated with contempt. Nothing we see or read in the media can be completely objective. The media can use stereotypes carelessly. But we need to demand that the media be fair and balanced. To uncover underlying viewpoints in the media ask "Who benefits?" or "Who loses?" For example, who benefits if old people are portrayed as silly in a sitcom? Who loses if only whites are shown in a TV show? Answering these questions helps us teach our children to think critically about what they see and hear. That is a crucial lesson in a democratic society.

5. TV is in business to make money. Networks sell airtime to advertisers so they can run their commercials. Advertisers sell products to viewers. It's important to teach kids that commercial television is not "free" entertainment. Its primary purpose is to sell viewers to advertisers. Advertising doesn't invite us to buy this or that product, it teaches us to buy. We are made to feel dissatisfied without certain new products. A useful question to ask is "Who's making money from the news tonight?" or a particular sporting event or show. The point is not that making money is wrong but that almost everything we see and hear on TV is subject to influence by a profit motive.

Get Busy Outside the Home—and Away from the Television Set

Fortunately, you don't always have to be on the defensive—protecting, warning, advising—to nurture your daughter's healthy self-image. Look for activities and classes that offer your girls a different world than the one you're trying to avoid on television or in the common culture. Music, art, baby-sitting, or other forms of entrepreneurship, drama, dancing, reading, computer technology, or scholastic pursuits are great activities to help build girls'

Tips from Parents on Building Your Daughter's Positive Self-image

- "When I see a concerted effort at straightening her room, putting the laundry away, taking the dog out, I praise the effort, thank her, and tell her how much she is appreciated."
- "We encourage her to try new things, and we praise her highly at the things she excels at."
- "We make it a point to tell her not just that she is beautiful, but how smart she is and what a good friend she is."
- "We value her opinion."
- "I just try to tell her that a healthy body is beautiful no matter what size."
- "We do not shrug off her feelings. We address them."
- "We do not poke fun or criticize efforts she makes at self-expression."
- "I remind her how good a person she is, and how I like it that she does not feel the need to follow her peer group."
- "Spending time as a family and one-on-one is very important."
- "We kiss, cuddle, hold her hand; remind her that she is not alone in her struggles."
- "We tell her that she is just fine being herself."

self-esteem and distract them from an obsession over how they look. Sports participation is a terrific way for girls to learn to feel good about their bodies and appreciate the way their physique contributes to athletic prowess. Religious affiliation and participation also often seems to confer a more positive self-image and gives girls more confidence in their abilities to control their affairs and destiny.[13]

A wonderful way for you and your daughter to discuss and understand female stereotypes and how to overcome them is

---

Books and Magazines to Help Build a Healthy Self-image

- *Great Books for Girls: More than 600 Books to Inspire Today's Girls and Tomorrow's Women*, by Kathleen Odean (Ballantine, 1997).
- For information on forming a mother-daughter book club, see *The Mother-Daughter Book Club*, by Shireen Douglas (Harper-Perennial, 1997); and *100 Books for Girls to Grow On*, by Shireen Douglas (HarperPerennial, 1998).
- *The Girls' Book of Wisdom: Empowering, Inspirational Quotes from 500 Fabulous Females*, by Catherine Dee (Little, Brown, 1999).
- *Teen Voices* is a magazine dedicated to challenging media images of women and serving as a vehicle for change. Call 888-882-TEEN or visit www.teenvoices.com.
- *New Moon* is for girls age eight to fourteen that emphasizes content encouraging girls to be smart, brave, and self-assured. Call 218-728-5507; or write New Moon, PO Box 3587, Duluth, MN, 55803-3587. The web site is at www.newmoon.org.
- *Girl* is a teen magazine that emphasizes racial and size diversity. Call 212-328-0180 or visit www.girlzine.com.
- *American Girl* is a magazine for younger girls that encourages self-esteem. Call 800-845-0005 or visit www.americangirl.com.

through a mother-daughter reading group. Such groups have become very popular across the country. You can find an easy guide to start a group and only need a few other mother-daughter pairs to get going. You can select, among other topics, books about girls' opportunities. One of the best parts of a reading club is that it creates a setting for girls to speak out on issues before an audience of listening and interested parents.

Questions to Ask Your Doctor

- My daughter fusses over what to wear each morning, trying on different outfits and complaining that she hates how she looks in everything. Is this a symptom of a poor self-image?
- My daughter is of normal weight but insists that she is too fat. Will you show her a growth chart and reassure her about her body size?
- My daughter has started puberty and is rapidly gaining weight. How do I know if this excess weight is healthy or is the start of a weight problem?
- I am on a diet and am restricting my food choices. My daughter complains that if it's okay for me to diet then she should be able to also. How can I persuade her that dieting is not good for her?

Resources

- Girls Inc. offers many programs in the fight to help make every girl strong, smart, and bold. These include programs in sports, science and technology, and health. Call 212-509-2000.
- Melpomene Institute has produced a video called *Heroes: Growing Up Female and Strong* to help girls build self-esteem. The cost is $19.95 for the video or $24.95 for the video plus curriculum. Call 651-642-1951.

- *Positive Self-Talk for Children*, by Douglas Bloch (Bantam, 1994), offers good advice for helping children feel self-confident.
- The company that produces the popular *American Girl* books for girls ages seven to twelve has a series of publications to give pre-teen girls facts and advice to reinforce positive social and moral values. Included: *The Care and Keeping of You: The Body Book for Girls* (1998) and *Help! An Absolutely Indispensable Guide to Life for Girls* (1995). For a catalog of American Girl products call 800-845-0005.
- *Growing a Girl*, by Dr. Barbara Mackoff (Dell Publishing, 1996), is a helpful guide to nurturing your daughter's sense of self-worth and independence.
- *The Body Project: An Intimate History of American Girls*, by Joan Jacobs Brumberg (Random House, 1997), takes a scholarly look at our cultural emphasis on appearance and what this does to girls.
- Purple Moon is a company that makes interactive computer games for girls ages eight to twelve. The offerings include *Soccer Challenge*, which teaches lessons about teamwork, and *Secret Paths*, programs that teach about self-confidence.
- These are all smart guides to encouraging media literacy in your daughter: *Screen Smarts: A Family Guide to Media Literacy*, by Gloria DeGaetano and Kathleen Bander (Houghton Mifflin Co., 1996); *Stay Tuned! A Family Media Guide*, by G. Jane Murphy and Karen Tucker (Doubleday, 1996); and *The Smart Parent's Guide to Kids' TV*, by Milton Chen, Ph.D. (KQED Books, 1995).
- The Center for Media Literacy offers materials to help parents, including *Making the Media Work for You: Action Ideas for Families*, a handout for parents, parenting classes, and discussion groups that costs $2. *Parenting in a TV Age* is a Media Literacy workshop kit for parent groups that costs $21.95. You can order either of these and numerous other materials from the Center for Media Literacy, 4727 Wilshire Boulevard, Suite 403, Los

Angeles, CA 90010. Call 800-226-9494. The web site is www.medialit.org.

- MediaWatch, a nonprofit organization dedicated to challenging biases in commercial media, offers information and resources. Visit www.mediawatch.com or call 831-423-6355.
- The publishers of *New Moon* magazine for girls offers a newsletter for parents to give examples and ideas on raising girls; *New Moon Network: For Adults Who Care About Girls*, Visit: www.newmoon. com or call 218-728-5507.
- About Face is a media literary organization focusing on the impact of media on the physical, mental, and emotional well-being of girls. It offers suggestions for raising awareness, resources, and information. Visit www.about-face.org.

CHAPTER 5

Fitness and Weight Control: Off the Scales and on to the Playground

I WORRY ABOUT my weight," says Shelley, fourteen. "I was always too heavy. But in junior high, I started getting really conscious about my weight because I was getting older. I wanted to lose weight so that guys would look at me. I started going on diets. But I could never stick to them. After a while, I got sick of it. I was trying to be something I wasn't. I'm trying to be happy with who I am right now. But I still look in the mirror at times and say, 'Dang, you know, I'm ugly.' "

Shelley's heartbreaking words describe a situation facing far too many of our daughters—the excruciating struggle with extra pounds. It's ironic that the growth of modern medicine ranks as one of the great achievements of the twentieth century and yet many of our children may someday go to their doctors with a completely preventable and often incurable health problem: obesity. The proof is in the numbers. Obesity affects one in five children; a rate that has doubled in the last two decades.[1] And, as Shelley's comments indicate, obesity is not just a physical health problem; it also wreaks havoc with a girl's self-esteem.

Children are getting fatter across all sex, age, racial, and ethnic groups with poor and minority kids, who often don't have as much access to recreational opportunities, being the most at risk. African Americans, Mexican Americans, Puerto Ricans, Native Hawaiians, and some Native Americans have very high rates of childhood obesity. Marcella, whose parents were born in Mexico, knows that she is too heavy but has found little support and help for achieving a healthier weight. "My mom, my dad, my aunts, my uncles, my brothers, my grandparents—they are always telling me I should go on a diet. When my grandpa came to town, I got bagged on for a month. My nickname in the family is 'Gordita.' It hurts when the criticism comes from your family; being called names by your family."

Why is this happening to our children? How can we be helpful and supportive without damaging a girl's self-esteem? Since the number of obese adults is rising, too, there is a suggestion that children are learning poor eating and exercise habits from adults. And there is another intriguing clue. Surveys show that U.S. children have not increased their caloric intake over the past several decades—that is, they do not seem to be eating more.[2] Thus, the most likely culprit in the obesity epidemic is the decline of physical activity and exercise. Indeed, if you look around, how many children do you see playing outdoors for hours, as many of us did as children? And, in most states, physical education classes have been dramatically cut back as more emphasis is shifted to basic academic skills.

The Goal: A Healthy Weight

While weight is an important determinant in health, what's also important is how you got there. In other words, if your child is slender but got there by vomiting after dinner, that's not a healthy weight. If your child is plump or even obese but has had a medical evaluation, is eating healthily along with the other family members, and is exercising vigorously several times a week, that is healthy—even if the child continues to weigh too much. Today we know that the key to weight control is to avoid dieting; eat normal, nutritious food; exercise regularly; avoid too many sedentary activities; and adopt the attitude that your body is precious at any size.[3] This approach will not ensure that every woman is thin. But it will be the foundation for strong health habits and a good body image.

This is a fairly new idea and is only beginning to seep into the adult culture. Indeed, it will take a major effort on the part of parents to teach their daughters this new paradigm. Most girls, some as young as seven, have already embraced the ideal of thinness through food restriction. Listen to Britteny, age thirteen:

> "I was always told by my friends and family that I was chunky and that I ate too much. They would say, 'Brit, if you just lost a few pounds, you would look so pretty and you would be happier.' Well, I took those words to heart and started dieting like crazy. But I felt like I wasn't losing enough, for no one commented on how great I looked. So I figured I was still too heavy. I exercised seven days a week, running three miles every day and eating less and less for many painful months. Still, the happy comments that I longed to hear weren't there. So I figured I need to lose more and more. Today I am thin, though I still feel very fat. But I think I can afford to be thinner. Because thinness equals happiness."

When girls become overly concerned with their weight and dieting, they risk adopting disordered eating patterns. The rise in childhood obesity is accompanied by a rise in eating disorders among girls. Annie, the mother of four girls ages eight, ten, twelve, and sixteen knows intuitively that dieting is closely tied to disordered eating. So she watches herself whenever the D word is mentioned. "I do not believe in diets for children because I think that could lead to eating disorders, which is a big fear of mine! Occasionally, they will show concern for their weight, but I try to downplay it. I explain what they could do if it really bothers them, but let it go after that."

But in many girls, especially during adolescence, body weight and fitness are appearance issues rather than health issues. "I'm always concerned about my weight," groans Grace, age nine. "Mom says it's normal, but I'm only a fourth grader and I'm eighty pounds. My figure is fine, and I look fine in a bathing suit. I just think I'm too heavy." Kids also fail to get the link between healthy eating and weight. One study found that the high priority teens attached to weight control was accompanied by the absence of caring about healthy eating.[4] Kids will restrict their calories, and will even exercise sometimes. But they do not see nutrition as a key factor in their health and body size.

Dieting is epidemic in our culture in virtually all age groups but the very young and the very old. In a 1992 survey of ninth through twelfth graders, 23.1 percent of males and 58.7 percent of females were attempting to lose weight at the time of the survey.[5] Many girls are imitating the weight patterns and concerns of their mothers. Jessica was a healthy, solid-looking child. But by age nine it was clear to her mother, Joan, that Jessica would be prone to the same problem that had plagued Joan since her adolescence: the big bones and solid physique that ran in the family also seemed to attract lots of unnecessary pounds. Jessica, while not seriously overweight, had developed heavy thighs and a thick

Caring About Health

This survey of 5,040 kids, ages 12 to 17, shows the percentage who felt their peers cared a lot about a particular health issue. While girls obviously cared about their weight, few cared about eating healthy.

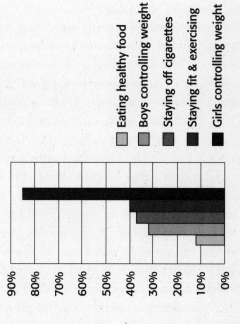

- Eating healthy food
- Boys controlling weight
- Staying off cigarettes
- Staying fit & exercising
- Girls controlling weight

waist. But what worried Joan more than anything was that Jessica loved food, especially her cooking. And Joan dreaded seeing her daughter start on the same endless round of dieting that she herself was still bound to. "I kick myself now for talking about how fat I am and how I need to lose weight," says Joan, a former executive secretary who is now a stay-at-home mom. "I couldn't bring myself to mention the word diet to Jessie. I didn't want her to start obsessing about her body the way I do about mine. She's just a kid." Nevertheless, Joan was concerned about her daughter's excess pounds—and rightly so.

Studies show, however, that dieting rarely works.[6] While some weight loss of five to ten pounds can often be managed and maintained in adults, losing a lot of weight is not only hard to accomplish, it's even harder to keep off. And dieting not only often fails, there is good evidence that it contributes to depression in girls. A study of eighty-three teenagers found that those who dieted were much more unhappy than a similar group of girls who didn't diet.[7] The harder it was for a girl to lose weight, the unhappier she became. Lilly, fifteen, is a girl who is dieting—and miserable. "I'm kinda afraid to step on the scale because I don't want to know how much I weigh. I feel like I'm overweight, so I don't eat that much—maybe once a day. I hear all the time about how you can get really sick if you don't eat. But what do I do if I don't feel like eating? When I do try to eat, I feel sick to my stomach."

While dieting is clearly unhealthy for girls, it's still important to try to avoid being overweight; not necessary for appearance, as our daughters would believe, but because being overweight is one of the single most damaging factors that control our long-term health. How then, do parents accomplish the seemingly conflicting goals of weight control while not obsessing over food? The answer lies in focusing on healthy eating and exercise habits. Even when a child develops a weight problem, the goal should continue to be the same: Eat normal and nutritious foods and exercise.

What Causes Obesity in Children?

Preventing obesity begins by understanding why it occurs. One or more of the following factors is probably involved.

Genes: There appears to be a genetic component to obesity. When children are obese, there is about a 30 percent chance both parents are obese.[8] But clearly genes don't explain the surge in obesity rates in the past twenty years. And, in about 25 to 35 percent of cases of child obesity, the parents are of normal weight.[9]

Eating habits: High-fat diets, heavy snacking, and overeating contribute to obesity. As many as 45 percent of all children snack on high-fat, calorie-dense foods at least twice a day.[10] Sometimes it's not the food but the way a family handles food that contributes to weight gain. We now know that children can regulate their own food intake and that parental control or interference ("Clean your plate, young lady" or "just one more bite") can thwart a child's ability to develop self-control. Children need to learn their own hunger and satiation cues. Parents should place balanced, healthy meals before a child and let her decide what and how much to eat. It's normal for young children in particular to eat a little at one meal and a lot at another.

The American College of Sports Medicine makes these recommendations to prevent and treat obesity:

- Children older than five years and adolescents should limit fat to no more than 30 percent of their daily caloric intake.
- Children and adolescents should eat more fruits, vegetables, and grains in their regular diet, and adequate amounts of lower-fat dairy products.

Exercise Forgotten as More Girls Diet

Girls' priorities about how to control their weight are often confused. Far too many diet while too few exercise.

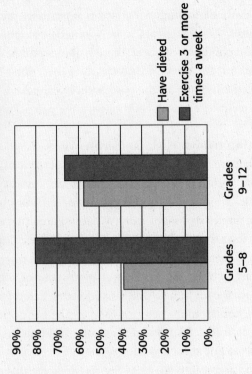

Grades 5–8

Grades 9–12

☐ Have dieted

■ Exercise 3 or more times a week

Source: The Commonwealth Fund survey of the Health of Adolescent Girls, 1997.

- In general, snacking should be less frequent. Snacks should include more healthy, low-fat choices such as fruits and vegetables and less of the high-fat, calorie-dense foods.
- Smaller portion sizes of nutritious foods should be consumed.

Sedentary lifestyle: Sitting before a television for hours (hours that could be spent in some physical activity) is often blamed for the rise in obesity in children. And you can add video games and computer use to the television as magnets that now draw children into sedentary lifestyles. One survey found that two out of three parents say their youngsters don't get enough activity because of lack of interest or competition from TV, video games, and computers.[11] Parents often inadvertently set the stage for sedentary behavior by actually encouraging it in their young children. Many parents can relate to Yvonne, the mother of two girls, ages six and four. "I've been trying to seriously limit the amount of TV my kids watch lately, although that's been hard. It was very easy to just plug them into a show—or two or three— so that I can get some work done."

Watching TV appears harmful to children in many ways (which we'll see in several other chapters). A 1998 study of kids ages eight to sixteen found that the more TV they watched, the greater the odds that they would be sedentary and overweight.[12] It's estimated that 60 percent of child obesity can be linked to excessive television watching. Simply reducing TV time may help a pudgy child to lose weight. One fascinating study compared a group of second and third graders who were given classroom instruction on why too much TV is harmful and an ordinary group of their peers.[13] The students who received the instruction reduced their TV-viewing time. And, by the end of the school year, the average kid in the instruction group gained nearly two pounds less than the average child in the normal group.

Studies have also linked long hours watching TV with the

increased consumption of foods advertised on TV. A typical child sees 10,000 TV advertisements for food each year, 95 percent of which are for sugared cereals, fast food, soft drinks, and candy.[14] Think of how many times your daughter has asked you to purchase some new snack food or cereal she's seen on TV.

Watching Your Child's Weight

While it's crucial not to nag children about their eating habits and instill a fear of food in them, it is appropriate to be concerned if your daughter appears to be too heavy. The consequences of obesity are profound in childhood for both health and psychosocial reasons. Obesity in childhood increases the risk of health problems in adulthood, including certain types of cancer, heart disease, arthritis, gallbladder disease, sleep apnea, and osteoarthritis. But obesity can cause health problems even during childhood. Obese children, it was recently shown, are increasingly being diagnosed with adult type of diabetes (type 2, known as adult-onset), which is the sixth-leading cause of death among diseases in the United States.[15] Children, if they develop diabetes, often have type 1, or juvenile diabetes, in which, for no known reason, the pancreas stops producing insulin. In type 2, the pancreas produces insulin but the organs grow increasingly resistant to it. If left untreated, it can cause serious damage to blood vessels.

> "My good friend is overweight. People make fun of her for this, and it really bothers her. She doesn't eat a lot, but doesn't exercise a lot, either. I want to help her and thought we could swim together every night. It would get us both in shape. But she was afraid someone would see her in her bathing suit at the pool."
>
> —Ashley, eleven

Obesity can also cause social misery for kids. Overweight kids are sometimes picked on or socially shunned. Even teachers may expect less of them academically or creatively because of their appearance. Obese children are apt to be viewed as more mature and may be faced with social situations inappropriate for someone their age. Obese children do not necessarily have a negative or low self-esteem because they pay close attention to their parents' remarks, which indicate love and acceptance of them.[16] But once a child reaches adolescence, her attitude often changes because she starts listening to cultural messages that tell her only thin is "in." Overweight teens often lose self-esteem and become depressed.

What to Do If Your Daughter Is Overweight

Any parent who thinks his or her daughter should lose weight should first consult an expert in childhood obesity. In younger children, it's difficult to assess a weight problem because kids grow at different rates and a chubby child may catch up in height later. As Suzanne, the mother of three girls, ages seven, ten, and thirteen, says: "My youngest two girls are a little overweight. But my oldest was also pudgy, until this year when she grew five inches in no time. I have faith that the younger two will do the same." If a child is still overweight at age eleven, however, she is likely to continue to have a weight problem. Getting expert advice to help your child is a must in order to try to help the child without creating new problems such as a fear of food, obsession with dieting, eating disorders, poor self-esteem, or other problems related to focusing on weight. Experts can best advise you and support your family during what will be a challenging family project. There are no easy solutions to addressing weight problems in children.

Weight-loss programs, even those that seem successful in

adults, have a poor track record in children and some experts believe, even exacerbate other problems, such as lack of confidence and self-esteem.[17] Some weight-control programs work, but they appear to work a whole lot better when the parents undergo counseling on how to model good eating behavior, prepare nutritious foods, and get their kids to exercise.[18] This is sometimes called behavioral, family-based treatment.

The Fitness Component

Carl is divorced from his wife, Erina. Although the two get along well, they don't see eye-to-eye on their seven-year-old daughter's weight. "My wife worries about Lindsay's weight. But I feel she'll grow into any extra weight she has," says Carl. "I am especially concerned that she doesn't start to worry about her weight at this tender age of seven. I promote exercise by introducing her to every sport and activity I can. I am an avid hiker, camper, skier, and biker, and I try to let her see me doing it. We talk about how running around and playing with the dog is good exercise, too."

One of the most important health lessons you can teach your daughter is that exercise isn't a mere option, like whether or not to go shopping at the mall on Saturday morning. Exercise is necessary for weight control, to keep bones and muscles strong, to keep the heart and lungs functioning at their best, and to help reduce normal stress and tension. Exercise has also been shown to lower the risk of certain types of cancers, diabetes, and hypertension. The rate of physical activity in our girls, however, is abysmal. According to the American College of Sports Medicine, less than half of children engage in routine physical activity.[19]

"It is very important for women to exercise because they enjoy it and not use exercise as a punishment. I try to separate exercise from the weight-loss process and urge women to pursue physical activity for their health, fitness, and self-esteem."

—Susan Calvert Finn, author, *ADA's Guide to Women's Nutrition for Healthy Living*

"I love to exercise. It makes me feel good inside and losing weight that very moment. I ride and walk a mile every day," enthuses Gloria, age ten. It's natural for children and preteens to be active and full of energy. According to several studies, however, natural play in children begins to drop at about age eleven.[20] By the first year of high school, most American girls have all but adopted sedentary lifestyles. Why should you be concerned if your daughter is not physically active? Parents may not worry about a girl's loss of interest in running, jumping, and sports around the time of puberty, especially if a girl is of normal weight and is healthy. But there are many reasons to be concerned about the decline in physical activity as our daughters grow up.

- A sedentary lifestyle may eventually contribute to weight gain in adulthood.
- Sedentary lifestyles are linked to an increased risk of physical injury. For example, an individual's first attack of back pain often occurs between the ages of six and fourteen years old. The majority of back pain occurs due to lack of muscular endurance, strength, and flexibility.
- Sedentary behavior in children (defined in one survey as fewer than two days of light or no exercise and no days of hard exercise) is associated with tobacco and marijuana use, lower fruit and vegetable consumption, and other negative health behaviors.[21]

Girls Exercise Less

The level of physical activity in both boys and girls peaks around 10th grade as this chart showing average hours per week of activity shows. But in every grade, girls are significantly less active.

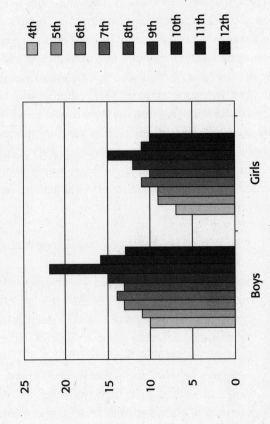

Boys   Girls

Legend: 4th, 5th, 6th, 7th, 8th, 9th, 10th, 11th, 12th

Source: International Life Sciences Institute, 1997.

Meanwhile, the benefits of exercise are great:

- Exercise during childhood and adolescence lowers blood pressure in adolescents with high blood pressure.
- Exercise increases good (HDL) cholesterol.
- Exercise increases bone density.
- Exercise has a positive effect on mood and lowers stress and anxiety.
- In girls, exercise may favorably alter the production of the hormones estrogen and progesterone during menstrual cycles in ways that contribute to a decreased risk of cervical, uterine, and breast cancer. Vigorous exercise can delay the onset of menstruation in girls, also decreasing lifetime estrogen exposure and possibly lowering the risk of breast cancer. In 1994, the National Journal of the Cancer Institute found that young women who exercised four hours a week reduced their breast cancer risk by 60 percent.[22]

"There are two main reasons why kids should exercise or pursue more physical activities," says Dr. James Sallis, an expert on child fitness. "To be healthy as kids and to increase the probability that they will remain physically active as adults." He recommends that kids spend some time each day involved in physical activity (games, sports, recreation, walking to school) and engage in vigorous activity at least three times a week for half an hour.

Motivating Your Daughter to Be Physically Active

"In high school, I looked around and started seeing girls wearing spaghetti straps and tank tops. I was wearing my mom's old pants. Then I noticed the girls on the drill team and what good shape they were in. I decided right then to start exercising," says Yolanda, fifteen.

By high school, many overweight girls will attempt to start exercise to help control weight. Many become frustrated at the difficulty that such effort takes. Parents will have the best chance of establishing an exercise ethic in their daughters if they start at a young age and link physical activities with fun. One survey found that the most common reason kids gave for being active is because it's fun.[23] "I have an eight-year-old daughter and I worry about her weight," says Judy. "She has a tendency to gain weight. It is so difficult to be a child these days. I don't want anyone to have any additional reasons to tease her. I don't tell her that she can't eat certain things, but I do encourage her to eat less fatty things. She plays soccer with the town team, and while doing so she has lost some weight. She is just starting track and we'll see if the same thing happens there. She is by no means overweight, but all the signs are there."

Look for activities that your child seems to truly enjoy. Don't force sports or activities on kids when they despise those activities. Be creative. For example, consider community races. Most have a one-mile run-walk that kids can participate in. Or, purchase a backyard basketball hoop or monkey bars. Give activity gifts for birthdays and holidays.

It's okay to insist that a child pick an activity of their choosing and then demand that they pursue it. Go ahead and be the "sedentary police." The American Academy of Pediatrics recommends that children watch no more than one to two hours of TV a day. Set a rule on when the television can be turned on. Or make TV time contingent upon other, more important tasks being finished first, such as homework or outdoor playtime. For example, tell your daughter she can watch half an hour of television for every hour she plays outdoors. Don't allow your child to have a TV in her room. It will make regulating TV that much harder. Finally, don't forget about video games and computers. They are like TV in that a child is often sedentary for a long stretch of time. It may be useful to buy an inexpensive kitchen timer and keep it next to the computer. Have your child set the timer for one hour—or whatever you think is suitable—and shut off the computer when her time is up.

Another proven factor in keeping kids active as they grow up is making the exercise ethic a family value. Parents' habits—Dad's especially—tend to influence children's activities. Dads who only enroll their boys in organized sports or prod their sons to go out and shoot hoops but do not extend these same invitations to their daughters do a double disservice. Not only is your girl not getting needed exercise and gaining confidence in her physical abilities, she is getting the message from you that only boys need to or should be physically active. Children (especially girls, some studies have found) whose parents are physically active are nearly six times as likely to be active than children whose parents are both inactive.[24]

It's important to start young in encouraging exercise because, by the adolescent years, a girl's friends will influence how active she is. But, again, parents can have a role in that by encouraging their daughter to stay true to her own interests and choose friends who embrace the same values and activities that she embraces.

Why Kids Shun Exercise

What can parents do with a daughter who hates breaking a sweat? First, it may be worthwhile to explore whether anything in her environment contributed to this attitude. Are the women in the family excessively feminine and not experienced in physical activity? Are your daughter's friends overly involved in boys, clothes, and makeup? The deeply imbedded cultural traditions that have long relegated women to the sidelines may still be influencing our daughters.

It's also worthwhile to question whether a school physical education program has turned your daughter off on anything having to do with the word physical. Studies show that kids who say they hate sports may have adopted that attitude in school. Nari, thirteen, is one of those kids. "I have mixed feelings about exercising," she says. "I enjoy some types of it. I don't enjoy one basic thing done *over* and *over* again. I like a mix of different types of exercise, liking running one day and aerobics next or a sport or something."

Unfortunately, some school PE programs focus too extensively on athletic accomplishment, leaving less athletically skilled children feeling embarrassed or bad about themselves. At other times, PE class is simply boring or seems irrelevant to kids.

Besides cultural traditions and hating PE, there are other reasons that our girls aren't getting enough exercise. Parents' lack of time to provide their kids with exercise opportunities is a common problem. Another reason families may spurn community sports programs is because of the emphasis on competition. While many communities do a good job of offering softball, baseball, basketball, soccer, golf, tennis, skating, swimming, and

FACT: Parents can't depend on school physical education classes to provide their kids with a daily dose of exercise.[25] Only one-third of schools offer PE classes. And according to one survey of kids who had PE in school, the classes accounted for, at best, less than one and three-quarter hours of physical activity per week.[26] If you are dissatisfied with the amount or quality of your child's physical education, let your school board know that you think it should be a priority. Another option is to work within your school to coordinate a group of parent volunteers who will run organized sports games at recess and will encourage all kids to participate.

other activities to girls, many of these are in the form of competitive leagues. Some girls are not cut out for competition and eventually drop out rather than be forced to compete at levels they are uncomfortable with. This is a problem that needs to be addressed by parent volunteers who want their unskilled or unathletic girls to have exercise opportunities in a suitable setting. Lobby for recreational, noncompetitive programs in your community. "There's nothing wrong with softball and football programs, but they don't serve the needs of all kids," says one exercise expert.[25]

The American Council on Exercise recommends these tips to get children physically active on a regular basis:

- You can't just tell your kids that exercise is fun—you have to show them. Get off the couch and go biking, rock climbing, or in-line skating with your kids. Skip rope or shoot baskets with them. Even if it's cold outside, encourage outdoor activities like skiing, hiking, or just playing in the snow.
- Invite your kids to participate in vigorous household tasks such as tending the garden, shoveling snow, or raking leaves. Demonstrate the value of these chores as quality physical activity.
- Plan outings and activities that involve some walking, like a trip to the zoo or a nature trail hike—even a trip to the mall.
- Set an example for your kids and treat exercise as something that should be done on a regular basis—like brushing your teeth or cleaning your room.
- Create a reward system to motivate your kids to move. For example, add a dollar or two to their weekly allowance for doing some kind of physical activity at least three days out of the week. Or recognize their fitness habits by purchasing a soccer ball, jump rope, or even in-line skates—anything that will keep them moving.
- Concentrate on the positive aspects of exercise. It can be a chance

Girls Don't Realize How Much Exercise They Need

Girls are significantly less active than boys,
yet just as many girls said they got enough exercise.

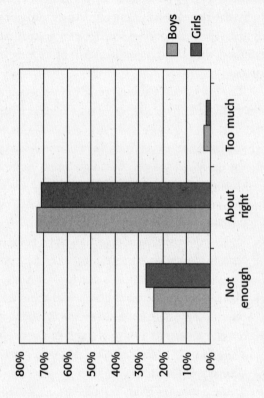

for the family to have fun together. Avoid competition, discipline, and embarrassment—these can turn good times into bad times. Praise your children for trying and doing.

- Keep in mind that kids are not always naturally limber. Their muscles may be tight and vulnerable to injury during growth spurts that occur during the elementary years. Be sure to include stretching as part of their fitness activities.
- Exercise and nutrition go hand in hand. Instead of high-calorie foods and snacks, turn your kids on to fruits and low or nonfat foods.

There are many other ways to get your daughter moving. Look for one of the growing number of kids' programs in sports and fitness clubs nationwide. Get your daughter on a bicycle as soon as she expresses interest. Make sure the bike fits, even if it means getting a new one every year or two (look for neighbors or friends to trade with). Kids can also be introduced to roller skates (with safety equipment), and swim lessons are a must, not just to teach a love of water sports but for safety reasons. If your child shows signs of being nonathletic, all the more reason to start young and try to teach some skills so she will build confidence. Practice throwing and catching a ball with your child, riding a bike, or jumping rope. "Both my kids are heavily involved in sports," says Chris. "The main thing is just to be there and give them attention. A hike or walk together is great, too." Here are some other tips for girls at different ages.

Age Six to Seven

Don't assume they're getting enough exercise just because they have lots of energy. You have to purposefully put it into a child's day. Dr. Laura Walther Nathanson notes in her book *The Portable Pediatrician's Guide to Kids* that even at age six, the boys at school and in the neighborhood tend to take over the play equipment and fields and girls tend to settle into quiet activities.

"Little girls who like to play quietly with dolls, books, and crafts are often left to their own preferences. Because they don't play actively, they aren't skilled at playing actively, and what starts out as a preference for one kind of play becomes a deliberate, strong avoidance of the other kind of play. Even little girls who enjoy active games can feel a great deal of pressure from their classmates to join them in the dollhouse corner," says Nathanson. She says it becomes harder as these girls grow up to get them active.

Age Seven to Eight

Ages seven and eight are crucial years in a kid's self-perception of her physical abilities, Nathanson says. She advises that this age is the last, best chance a chubby girl has of slimming down by growing in height and slowing down in weight gain.

Age Nine to Eleven

If your child isn't moving yet, try an activity in which it's acceptable to be unskilled or a beginner, such as soccer, swimming, tennis, or ice-skating. Have your child participate with a friend. Get some coaching. Make sure kids know you feel exercise is important. You do this by planning activities for them or ways for them to be active and suggesting physical activities when you tell them to turn off the computer or TV.

Preteens

Watch for that vulnerable stage when your daughter and her friends may be turning their attention to clothes and boys and thinking less about exercise. A look at most community recreational leagues, such as softball leagues, shows a large drop-off in participation between the ages of ten and twelve. If your daughter wants to quit an activity, press hard for an explanation and encourage her to stay in the activity or ask her to choose another one. It's okay to tell your daughter she simply cannot be sedentary and has to pursue a regular physical activity of her choice.

Teenagers

For teens whose metabolisms are shifting into adult metabolisms, it's time to pick up the pace of exercise a bit. The goal should be aerobic activity at least four times a week. Aerobic means heavy breathing, perspiring, and an increased heart rate. Adding music or TV might increase the teen's participation. If you have a home bike, treadmill, or some other home gym equipment, consider stationing it before a TV and allow your daughter to watch her favorite programs while working out. But don't purchase any extra equipment until your teenager has broken sedentary habits and a regular activity pattern is established. Be aware that the major obstacles in getting teen girls to exercise tend to be time constraints, disinterest, boredom, or difficulty breaking established sedentary habits.

Questions to Ask Your Doctor

- Is my child's weight appropriate for her height?
- Are there any indications that my child is gaining too much weight for her height and age?
- Can I obtain a referral to consult with a nutritionist about my family's nutrition and eating habits? (Sometimes, a doctor referral will pave the way for insurance reimbursement for consultations with a registered dietitian.)
- Can you refer me to a fitness program specifically for children who are overweight?
- Is a walking program helpful or does my child need to break a sweat in order to accelerate weight loss?

- I was plump as a child, but around age ten I shot up several inches and my weight was fine. Can I expect the same thing to happen to my child?
- I serve my family healthy meals but my twelve-year-old daughter, who is overweight, sneaks snack foods into her room. What should I do to prevent this?

Resources

- American Dietetic Association: 800-366-1655.
- President's Council on Physical Fitness and Sports: 202-609-9000.
- University-based pediatric obesity programs can be found at www.niddk.nih.gov/health/nutrit/nutrit.htm.
- In 1998, the U.S. Department of Health and Human Services Maternal and Child Health Bureau released guidelines for practitioners for the evaluation and treatment of overweight children. For reprints contact: the National Maternal and Child Health Clearinghouse, 2070 Chain Bridge Road, Suite 450, Vienna, VA 22182–2536.
- For the brochure *10 Tips to Healthy Eating and Physical Activity for You*, geared to kids ages nine to fifteen, send a SASE to P.O. Box 65708, Washington, D.C. 20035.
- For the brochure *Helping Your Overweight Child*, published by the Weight-Control Information Network and the National Institute of Diabetes and Digestive and Kidney Diseases, send a business-size SASE to 1 Win Way, Baltimore, MD 20892–3655. Or call 301-951-1120.
- Several helpful books for girls to encourage exercise and a healthy body image are: *The Right Moves: A Girl's Guide to Getting Fit and Feeling Good*, by Tina Schwager and Michele Schuerger (Free Spirit Publishing Inc., 1999) and *Body Pride: An Action Plan for Teens Seeking Self-Esteem & Building Better Bodies*, by Cynthia

Stamper Graff, Janet Eastman, and Mark C. Smith (Griffin Publishing Group, 1997).

- The Federal Department of Health and Human Services offers an exercise and nutrition program guide for black girls and women entitled *Sisters Together: Move More, Eat Better Program Guide*. To obtain the guide call the Weight-Control Information Network, at 301-951-1120 or visit www.niddk.nih.gov/health/nutrit/win.htm. Ask for NIH Publication No. 99–3329.

CHAPTER 6

Sports and Athletics:
Playing Catch-up

UNTIL she was a sophomore, nothing too spectacular had happened to fifteen-year-old Emily. Her family, recent immigrants to the country, struggled to make ends meet on low wages. And Emily felt that she was no beauty and had no special talents. But that was before a track coach noticed her strength and coordination during a gym classes and urged her to try out for the team. Emily's eyes brighten when she talks about sports.

"I like the competition. It makes me feel good about myself. I like working out, even lifting weights. And when I win I get really happy because I make my parents and brother proud. When I got my awards and my letter last year, they were really proud. That's what I like the most."

It wasn't that long ago when girls like Emily lacked the opportunity to find fulfillment through sports participation. Clearly, much has changed in the world of women's sports. A generation ago, girls had limited chances to flex their muscles. Indeed, you may remember all too well how few girls' sports were offered when you were growing up—before the passage of Title IX legislation in 1972 barred sex discrimination in schools sports programs and other areas. You may even see the opportunities available to their daughters today with some envy! "Back then there were some sports available to girls but they weren't encouraged," says Sandy, the mother of a nine-year-old girl who enthusiastically pursues a different sport every season.

While there is great progress, there are still more girls not participating routinely in sports than there are enthusiasts. Girls account for only 37 percent of all high school athletes.[1] Moreover, there are still many things we don't know about the effect of sports on girls' lives. There are still many barriers to their participation. And we still don't see the majority of girls growing up with at least some basic sports skills. Nevertheless, stories like Emily's should compel parents to explore sports as a way to enrich their daughters' mental, physical, and emotional lives.

How Sports Participation Benefits Girls

Girls in sports are fit and more in tune with their bodies compared to sedentary girls. They learn more about nutrition due to their desire to understand how eating properly will help them in athletic performances. They are satisfied and feel in control of their bodies and can utilize the strength and endurance that comes naturally to them. Girls in sports tend to place a priority on their own needs and interests. They appear less susceptible to peer pressure and less concerned with what others think. They do not question the idea that girls can be feminine and can also put on a

Participation in Girls Sports

A comparison of these surveys taken seven years apart shows more involvement among young girls but little changes among girls ages 12 to 17.

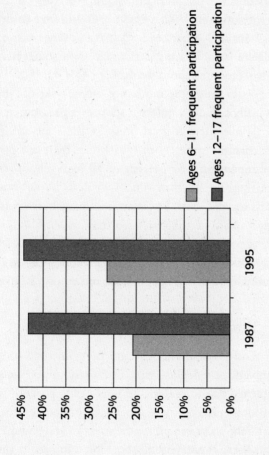

Ages 6–11 frequent participation

Ages 12–17 frequent participation

Source: Sporting Goods Manufacturing Assn.

uniform and work up a sweat on the basketball court. Jane's daughter, Amber, thirteen, swims and rides a bike to stay active year-round. But she also looks forward to softball season each spring. "Softball has taught her many, many things: cooperation, encouraging teammates who aren't as experienced as she is, good sportsmanship, time management, and how to set one's mind to doing something—like learning to hit—and doing it," says Jane.

Girls in sports are also more likely to stay in school and go to college. And many studies have documented the physical and mental health benefits to girls in sports.[2]

- Reduces girls' risk for obesity and hyperlipidemia (high levels of cholesterol), which can then reduce the risk of heart disease and certain cancers.
- Strengthens bones, reducing the lifetime risk of osteoporosis.
- Builds muscle strength.
- Reduces stress, tension, and depression.

Sports not only provide many long-lasting physical benefits, they offer unique social and emotional growth opportunities to girls. Girls in sports learn such life skills as how to communicate with peers and adults, support others, commit to a task, collaborate, make decisions, and deal with achievement and disappointment. They learn a work ethic and leadership skills that will serve them well in adult life. In fact, a survey of Fortune 500 companies showed that eight out of ten high-ranking women leaders reported that they were "tomboys" or "jocks" in their youth.[3]

"The physical strength, competence, and sense of mastery in sports help girls with what they're dealing with. They can make decisions from a point of strength. Boys make that assumption. Girls don't."
—Gloria Feldt, Planned Parenthood
Federation

There are many reasons why girls participate in sports, and each of them needs to be recognized and honored by parents. Many girls like the competitive thrill. Others are trying to get in shape. Some girls like the social aspect of team sports. Still others like the feeling of learning new skills and improving. Almost all girls like having fun. "I play soccer and basketball," says Jamie, ten. "I do it as an act of exercise and just to have fun with my friends. I like it because I like to have a fun thing to do during my spare time."

Why Girls Don't Play

Despite the clear advantages of playing sports, only about one-quarter of all girls ages six to eleven participate regularly.[4] Most girls don't grow up learning the basic skills of even a *single* sport.

There are several reasons for this. The most obvious is that some girls just don't like sports. They would much rather play quietly with dolls or toy ponies or would rather play the piano or paint pictures. Some lack coordination or strength that would help them do well at sports. Colette, the mother of two girls, has made a concerted effort to get Stephanie, fourteen, into a sport. "She won't participate unless forced," sighs Colette. "She's extremely thin, and this apparently reduces the motivation to exercise. She played basketball last year. She would probably disagree, but I think the social interaction, need for discipline, and exercise were the most important parts of the experience."

You should respect the choices of your daughter if she was born without the slightest urge to participate in sports. But it is still worth insisting that she at least try some sports and then allow her to quit if she doesn't enjoy them. Don't insist on a particular sport. Let your daughter have a choice in what sport she wants to try. Kurt has watched his daughter, Amy, nine, closely to gauge where her sports interests might lie. "My daughter is not very interested in organized team sports, like soccer, but the little boy who lives next door is. By seeing him play and getting a chance to go out and interact with other kids, she is getting interested in soccer. I'm thrilled. I have also enrolled her in roller-skating lessons, but I don't push her. I just let her have fun and play and, through that, she'll keep a positive attitude about activities."

If your daughter is unathletic, the earlier you try sports, the better chance you have for success. All girls at young ages, even the ones who will turn out to be great athletes, are beginners and lack skills. Your daughter will fit in at ages six, seven, and eight no matter who else is playing. Starting young appears important to the development of a lifelong appreciation of sports.[5]

Despite inroads girls and women have made in sports, there remains pervasive sexism in sports—some of it based on myth and misunderstanding. For example, the expression "throwing like a girl," which has long meant an awkward and inefficient throwing style, is both politically and biologically incorrect. If a person has underdeveloped muscles, a lack of instruction or experience, that person may throw poorly whether male or female.[6]

If your daughter seems naturally drawn to more traditionally feminine pursuits, look for physical activities with characteristics that may attract her for other reasons, such as skating with its pretty costumes or tennis with the cute outfits. Some completely nonsports-oriented girls may still enjoy ballet and other forms of dance, activities that provide many of the same benefits as organized sports.

Many high school–age girls benefit from the exercise involved in cheerleading. Shannon, sixteen, is a cheerleader, and her mother, Eileen, thinks the experience has been great for her daughter. "She gets a huge amount of exercise, learns coordination, and it really helps her self-esteem." Indeed, cheerleading nowadays also demands athletic skill, endurance, and strength. But there are some drawbacks to cheerleading that parents and their daughters should consider. First, cheerleading usually emphasizes body size, body image, and sex appeal to the extent that modern cheerleading uniforms often feature tight clothing and bare midriffs. And, while cheerleaders do work hard, their primary function is to cheer on competitive athletes (mostly the male athletes). Moreover, in some schools cheerleading has been used to satisfy a school's requirements under Title IX, the law that gives girls as many athletic opportunities as boys.[7] If cheerleaders are counted as athletes, that may mean a school can get away with not fielding a girls' soccer team, golf team, or some other girls' sport. "If cheerleading starts falling into an umbrella definition of sport, that means each time a girl becomes a cheerleader there is one less opportunity for another girl to be on a sport played in a national and international arena," says Donna de Varona, a former Olympic swimmer and a founder of the Women's Sports Foundation.

The final barrier to girls' participation in sports is the saddest. Too many girls who would love to play sports can't because of economic reasons or because their parents lack the time or ability to take their daughters to practices and games. Many poor girls, girls of color, and girls with disabilities have economic or environmental barriers that deter their participation.[8] (See Resources for information on free sports programs for girls and advice for girls with disabilities.) If your family cannot afford sports participation fees, look into after-school neighborhood programs like the YWCA and Girls Inc., which may have girls sports programs. In addition, many cities with recreation programs will admit any child regardless of the ability to pay. Look for soccer programs, in particular. While it is surely not easy for some poor families to have their children in sports, make a concerted effort on behalf of your daughter. The benefits she will gain by playing sports may well offset some of the disadvantages in her life.

Why Girls Quit

It's opening day for the girls' softball season in Orange, California. Girls dressed in bright uniforms with matching hair bows parade around the field carrying their team banner. There are a dozen or more teams of girls ages seven to ten. But the age twelve division is 50 percent smaller. And only a few teams make up the age fourteen division.

What's happening on this field in this town is representative of a disturbing trend everywhere. The big negative in the hype over the girls' sports trend is that girls drop out of sports at a rate six times that of boys.[9] The drop-out trend in girls sports is particularly apparent around the ages of twelve to fourteen. A look at recreational sports programs will show that many girls—with the exception of the more feminine sports of figure skating and gymnastics—begin to lose interest around the time of puberty. This is a disturbing phenomenon that adults should examine. Why do girls who love to slide into second base, muscle out competitors for rebounds, and slam hockey pucks into the net eventually become reticent about sports?

Part of the reason may have to do with society's expectations about how women behave. At puberty, girls begin to look more like women, and there may be lingering perceptions that *women* shouldn't get dirty or bruised in tough games. Parents or relatives may communicate this idea to girls even nonverbally by losing interest in their games, practices, and progress.

Another reason older girls may drop out of sports is due to a mistaken belief that female athletes are, or will become, lesbians.[10] This kind of homophobic myth has led many girls to worry about appearing too masculine for fear of being labeled a lesbian. There is also an unfounded belief among some parents that girls will be persuaded to become lesbians by participating in certain sports.

While many girls quit sports because of the lack of encouragement and support, some—incredibly—quit because too much is demanded of them. "Sometimes I think coaches take this stuff too darn seriously and expect the kids to not have a life outside of their sport," says Trina, the mother of two girls who play soccer. "Hey, they're just kids, and they need to have a well-rounded life." Girls as young as ten can be burned out as athletes. This usually happens to extremely talented girls who show immediate promise in a sport at a young age (and perhaps cause their parents to envision college athletic scholarships). It's tempting, with these young sports stars, to obtain private coaching, join all-star and travel teams, and compete year-round. But parents beware: The strategy can backfire if a child starts sensing she is losing her childhood to the quest of becoming a sports phenomenon.

Problems in Sports Participation

There can be too much of a good thing when it comes to sports. Increasingly, athletic participation is associated with illness, injury, and addiction to exercise.[11] For girls, one of the biggest threats is called the Female Athlete Triad. This is a set of inter-related problems that usually occur in very highly trained athletes. The triad tends to develop in sports in which an emphasis is placed on maintaining a constant, and often low, weight, such as dance, ice-skating, and gymnastics. But the problem can also occur in girls who pursue track, basketball, and other sports. The triad of problems consists of *eating disorders, amenorrhea,* (the absence of menstruation) and *osteoporosis.*

Eating disorders refers to a range of harmful and unnatural eating behaviors that girls employ in order to lose weight. They may force themselves to vomit after eating, eat only tiny amounts of food, or exercise excessively to burn off the calories they consumed. (For more on this topic, see chapter 8 on eating disorders.) Girls who participate in sports in which a lean body is emphasized are four times more likely to develop an eating disorder compared to girls in nonlean sports.[12] Patricia, sixteen, was one of those girls. She took laxatives in order to keep her weight down. "I think my sports participation fueled the eating disorder," she says, adding that she routinely ran ten miles a day while also starving her body of nutrients. Eating disorders do not result from participation in these sports but from psychological problems or issues in the girls who participate in the sports.

The second component, amenorrhea, means the absence of menstruation in a girl age sixteen or older who has developed other sex characteristics, such as breast development. When a girl's period has not started by this stage, the disorder is called primary amenorrhea. If a girl starts her period but then menstruation stops for three or more cycles, the diagnosis is secondary amenorrhea. Amenorrhea usually occurs because a girl has lost too much weight (due to an eating disorder or excessive exercise). The consequences of amenorrhea are related to the third component of the triad: osteoporosis.

Osteoporosis is a word that is usually associated with elderly women. But girls, tragically, can develop this condition when they have amenorrhea and are eating poorly. The loss of bone during adolescence is of particular concern because these are the years during which a girl should be banking extra bone to offset the inevitable loss of minerals later in life.

If your daughter is heavily involved in sports, you should be aware of the symptoms of the triad. Perhaps the best way to prevent the development of this problem, however, is to avoid putting any pressure on your daughter to lose weight. Moreover, girls should be educated about proper nutrition, safe training practices, and the warning signs that they may be pushing their bodies too hard.

Who Is at Risk for the Female Athlete Triad?

Potentially all physically active girls and women could be at risk for developing one or more components of the triad. The biological changes, peer pressure, societal drive for thinness, and body-image preoccupation that occur during puberty make adolescence the most vulnerable time. Participation in sports that emphasizes low body weight can also be a risk factor. Those sports include:

1. Sports in which performance is subjectively scored (dance, figure-skating, diving, gymnastics, aerobics)
2. Endurance sports emphasizing a low body weight (distance running, cycling, cross-country skiing)
3. Sports requiring body contour–revealing clothing for competition (volleyball, swimming, diving, cross-country running, cross-country skiing, track, cheerleading)
4. Sports using weight categories for participation (horse racing, some martial arts, wrestling, rowing)
5. Sports emphasizing a prepubertal body habitus for performance success (figure-skating, gymnastics, diving)

The Female Athlete Triad also occurs in nonathletes and in physically active girls and women who are not training or competing in a specific sport.

Source: American College of Sports Medicine.

Injuries

About 775,000 kids are seen in hospital emergency rooms each year for sports injuries.[13] Up to half of all injuries to children and adolescents are sustained while playing organized sports, reports the American College of Sports Medicine. Injuries are most likely to be musculoskeletal and occur from overuse or a single blow or twist.[14] Don't assume that because your daughter is young, injuries are improbable. Girls are particularly susceptible to injury because they are growing and many of the body's tissues, such as growth cartilage, are vulnerable to strain.[15] Injuries seem to be common during the peak growth spurt in adolescence, perhaps because of biochemical changes in the body during puberty. Girls may be at risk of overuse injuries because of the increase in body fat composition at puberty, the lack of increased muscle strength, and the changing alignment of the lower extremities.[10] Overuse injuries often occur in children who pursue a particular sport year-round. Participating in several different sports might help to make a child more physically well-rounded and less prone to injuries.

There are ways to curb these unnecessary injuries. For instance, caution should be taken during the months when your child is obviously having a growth spurt. A growth spurt usually means adding nine to ten pounds in a year or growing several inches.

Stretching exercises should be taught and encouraged as a prelude to every workout. The length or load of a workout should be curtailed. Some injuries are the result of microscopic strains and fractures that are never given a proper chance to heal and thus become a chronic, nagging problem. Let your daughter rest until soreness or pain has disappeared. Proper safety equipment should be used in all practices and games. Strength training has been shown to be helpful in kids to prevent injuries, providing that safety rules and guidelines are closely followed.[17]

Girls need to be especially aware of their tendency toward knee injuries. As the number of girls in sports has risen, so too has the rate of serious knee injuries in girls.[18] Females—especially those in basketball and soccer—appear to be almost four times as likely to suffer from a particular knee injury called the anterior cruciate ligament injury.[19] It's important to take seriously a girl's complaint about an injury. While many are minor and should not be the focus of excessive attention or coddling, neither is it appropriate to dismiss your daughter's injury as being "just part of the game." Many injuries do not get appropriate care due to this attitude. Another important component to keeping your daughter healthy is to have her undergo a sports examination six to eight weeks before starting a sport.

> "I just enjoy playing sports. I feel strong. I try to beat my own record. And it feels really good when I beat it."
>
> —Chrissy, fourteen, a high school swimmer

As more girls become involved in sports, there is some concern that they will pick up some of the bad habits that some of their male counterparts have already experienced. For example, you may assume steroids are something that only surface in gyms where body builders are honing 250-pound physiques. Not true. Even school-aged athletes are exposed to steroid use—girls as well as boys. Steroid use among girls has nearly doubled since 1991.[20] This phenomenon may be due to a trend among female athletes to develop a "hard" look, emphasizing highly toned muscles and leanness. But anabolic steroids and over-the-counter substances called hormone precursors (such as androstenedione) are extremely dangerous. They may cause heart and liver damage and could even cause reproductive problems in women.[21] Girls need to be told about the dangers of steroids because many prevention programs presently are aimed only at boys (who have twice the rate of steroid use). You should know the warning signs that your daughter may be using steroids. These include a sudden increase of lean muscle mass; a sudden improvement in performance; behavior that indicates an obsession with her body; hair loss; menstrual disruptions; or a deepened voice.

Parents should obtain a list of safety rules and safety equipment from coaches in order to ensure that girls minimize their risks. Items to look for include:

- A list of all required safety equipment and assurance that the equipment will be used in practices as well as games
- Safety equipment that fits the athlete and is not altered from its original condition or form
- Helmets, if required, that are rated according to the standards of a national institution
- Safety equipment that is maintained to function properly
- Shoes that are replaced when worn to the point where they have lost their protective functions
- Playing surfaces that are in good condition

Source: American College of Sports Medicine, "The Prevention of Sport Injuries of Children and Adolescents," 1993.

Adults

"The best experience is when there is someone other than the parent showing kids how to play, proper technique, etc.," says Jim, whose daughter, Kelly, is eleven. Many parents, like Jim, find that their kids resist taking instruction from a parent but will listen to another adult. Ideally, you should be supportive and leave the instruction to coaches. The role of coaches and parents is to instruct, provide support, and oversee a girl's safety. They are not contributing by belittling a girl, trying to force her to become something she isn't, or by overemphasizing winning. Much poor behavior on the part of adults comes because of the emphasis on competition. This all-too-real problem in organized youth sports has led Sherry to give up on sports for her daughter, Andrea, fourteen. "She is not into organized sports at all, and I have never encouraged it," Sherry says. "I do not like the politics and the parental involvement." Michael, another parent of girls, says this: "Mostly, the effects I see from organized sports are the ways my daughters are excluded and looked down upon by their peers because my daughters weren't good enough."

Competition should remain of secondary importance until at least the junior high school level. You should make sure that the coach teaching your daughter emphasizes safety above all else and exhibits appropriate values and behavior. Coaches should have positive attitudes and encourage girls to have fun while trying their best. When Leese, thirteen, experienced hostility from other players, her coach failed to step in and demand that the girls behave as teammates. The result was that Leese says she will probably never play sports again. "I used to play softball, but there were girls on my team who made fun of my weight. They said, 'It's too bad you can't play softball. You can't run.' They talked bad about me. I told my mom that I wanted to quit and she said don't worry about what other people say. But I started crying because I didn't want to play with those girls. After three months, I quit. I really loved softball."

Girls will have a good experience if adults use common sense about the need to be encouraging and helpful. Girls who have positive coaches have the best experience in sports, regardless of how well the girl or team performed competitively.

It's up to you to monitor practices and games and be prepared to transfer your daughter to another team or league or even (in serious situations) report a coach whose behavior concerns you. Julianne, twenty-four, has been an all-star athlete since she was eight. But, in hindsight, she regrets letting one particular coach have so much influence over her life. "I had a male coach throughout the most formative years of my training. I trusted him, got along well with him, and felt he shaped my athletic career. However, I had a relationship with another male coach and later found out that I was not the only one he had a relationship with. It started when I was very young and I have only now realized the power and manipulation a male coach can have over a young, female athlete."

You, too, should take a hard look at your own attitudes and

behavior regarding your daughter's sports participation. Remember that this activity is solely for your child's benefit. Be encouraging, empathetic, and low-key. Cheer, but never make critical comments to your child or berate your child during a performance. Emphasize that sports should be fun and that you're interested in seeing your daughter get exercise, develop new skills, learn how to interact in a team setting, and develop an appreciation for an activity that could provide a lifetime of enjoyment. Even if you lack interest in sports, try to be there for your daughter and let her know you are proud of her involvement.

Here are some other tips for parents:

- Emphasize fun. Kids generally don't care if they win, as long as they have a good time. Very young kids won't even care about the score.
- Don't start a too-shy or anxious child into a sport before she is ready. It may cause her to avoid sports altogether.
- Don't put your child in situations that are too difficult for her. Look for recreation programs that emphasize instruction for beginners and advance from that point, making sure your daughter isn't placed in a situation in which everyone else has more advanced skills than she does.
- Don't expect your child to have similar abilities as parents. Parents who find themselves envisioning an Olympic gold medal or a college athletic scholarship should take a hard look at why their child is in the sport and whether the activity is healthy.
- Tell your child what kind of behavior you expect of her. For example, you want her to have fun, listen to the coach, and obey team rules. Tell your child that you want to know if she dislikes the sport or is tired of it and would prefer to do something else.
- Watch for signs that your child is being overtaxed or may be injured. Kids may not say when they are hurt if they are afraid of disappointing their parents.

- Never dismiss an injury as insignificant if the child is hurting.
- Let your child select a sport and decide how involved she wants to be in it. For example, ask her if she would like to practice once a week or twice a week.
- Remember that socializing is part of the fun. If you recall the camaraderie, socializing, and goofing around that you enjoyed while participating in recreational sports, then perhaps you can better understand that your child probably likes the same things. Give your child the opportunity to enjoy the game without letting things get too serious.
- Keep an eye on your child's coach to make sure kids are kept safe and are respected.
- Be involved and interested. Your daughter's success in sports will have much to do with parents' involvement, support, and actual physical presence. Attend your child's games and practices.

Questions to Ask Your Doctor

- Is my child ready for organized sports?
- What safety equipment (including mouth and eye protection) do you recommend for her sport?
- How often should she undergo a sports physical?
- Is her school-sponsored sports physical (usually done at the school) adequate?
- My daughter tends to overtrain. What is a reasonable amount of practice or training for someone her age?
- My daughter wants to start lifting weights. Is this safe at her age and under what circumstances?
- My daughter's coach encourages his athletes to eat a particular diet. Is this okay?

Resources

- Center for Research on Girls & Women in Sport, 203 Cooke Hall, 1900 University Avenue S.E., University of Minnesota, Minneapolis, MN 55455; 612-625-7327; www.kls.coled.umn.edu/crgws/
- Parents whose kids resist sports might want to read this book for some good tips and a better understanding: *Why Johnny Hates Sports: Putting the Fun Back in Sports for Boys and Girls*, by Fred Engh (Avery Press, 1999).
- A free copy of "The Female Athlete Triad" position statement can be obtained by sending a business-size SASE to: American College of Sports Medicine, Public Information Department., c/o Triad, P.O. Box 1440, Indianapolis, IN 46206-1440.
- *Good Sports: The Concerned Parent's Guide to Competitive Youth Sports*, by Rick Wolfe (Sports Pub., 1996).
- *The Total Sports Experience for Kids: A Parent's Guide to Success in Youth Sports*, by Aubrey H. Fine and Michael L. Sachs (Diamond Co., 1997).
- This is a web site where kids can learn about various sports. It also features stories on major figures in sports and statistics: www.yahooligans.com/content/ka/almanac/sports/index.html.
- The Sports Illustrated for Kids web site has sports stories and news, trivia, and games: www.sikids.com/index.html.
- The Girl Power web site has stories about great women athletes and tips on how girls can improve their skills: www.health. org/gpower/girlarea/sports/index.htm.
- Just Sports for Women is a web site featuring sports news and information for older girls: www.justwomen.com/
- PE Central Sport web site has tips, drills, and resources in twenty-three sports: www.pecentral.org.
- *Sports Medicine for Parents and Coaches*, by Daniel J. Boyd, M. D. (Georgetown University Press, 1999).

- The Melpomene Institute has information and resources for girls in sports. 1010 University Avenue, St. Paul, MN 55104; 651-642-1951; www.melpomene.org/
- For information on how people with disabilities can become more involved with sports, request a free copy of *Research on Physical Activity and Disability: An Emerging National Priority.* Send a business-size SASE to: ACSM Public Information Department, P.O. Box 1440, Indianapolis, IN 46206-1440.
- Skyhawks is a business that offers a wide range of summer sports camps and helps to send economically disadvantaged youths when possible. It is located at P.O. Box 18529, Spokane, WA 99228-0529, or call 800-804-3509.
- Recommended reading about the difference sports can make in the lives of girls: *In These Girls, Hope Is a Muscle*, by Madeleine Blaise (Warner, 1996).

CHAPTER 7

Nutrition: A Diet for Now and Forever

I TRY TO EAT healthy at school," says Lauren, thirteen. "But at home, my aunt cooks because my mom works long hours. My aunt—she cooks everything with grease. So I say, oh well, and I just eat it."

It's not always easy to make sure your child is eating right. Surely, Lauren's parents want her to be healthy. But they, like many parents, find it hard to work good nutrition into hectic family schedules. And few adults grew up in homes where nutrition was emphasized the way it is today. (Did you ever hear your mother talk about saturated fat?) Girls like Lauren, however, are beginning to learn more about nutrition in school. And families need to support their kids' desires to eat healthy foods, even if it means breaking away from some traditional cooking methods and favorite family dishes.

Since eating habits, food preferences, and relationships with food are set early in life, it's important for you to consider just how you want your daughter to think about food. It may sound silly to talk about "thinking about food" and "relationships with food," but the high incidence of overeating, obesity, dieting, and disorder eating suggests that we Americans *do* have a lot of food issues and need to develop ways of eating that meet our nutritional needs and fit in with our lifestyles and social and cultural traditions. Learn the components of healthy eating, and then model them for your daughter. That may mean replacing some of the beliefs and practices that you grew up with. "A lot of parents look for convenience with food preparation. But all of a sudden, our kids are twenty-three years old and they're asked to be healthy. But they've already developed bad habits," says Dr. Bill Viand, a government researcher on nutrition.[1] Far better is it to teach kids proper nutrition and eating habits early in life. "When you're hooked early, it's difficult to change."

> "Nutrition is the single biggest factor influencing the health and well-being of women at any stage of life. Too often, however, nutrition is neglected, especially at critical times during a woman's life."
>
> —Susan Calvert Finn, The Journal of
> Women's Health

While diets vary widely among individuals, national surveys tend to show the following common patterns among American youths:

- Too high in fat and saturated fat. Studies show that the average child consumes 36 percent of her calories from fat.[2]

- Too high in cholesterol. More than 75 percent of children eat more cholesterol than is recommended.[3]
- Too high in salt. Most Americans, including children, eat double or triple the one teaspoon a day that is considered adequate.
- Too high in sugar.
- Frequent skipping of meals.
- Frequent snacking.
- Too low in fiber.
- Too low in calcium.
- Too low in folate, vitamin A, vitamin E, vitamin B6, iron, zinc, and magnesium.

"In recent years, we've discovered that a high-fat diet, which means eating relatively large amounts of meat, dairy products, and fried foods, is the main cause of atherosclerosis, coronary heart disease, stroke, certain forms of cancer, and obesity."

—Dr. Benjamin Spock

What a Healthy Diet Looks Like

In Shirley's family, "we stress the greens. We try to eat a lot of fruits and vegetables. We say good food first and foremost, and then you can have some junk here and there." Undoubtably, Shirley's daughter, Christy, fifteen, will benefit greatly from this simple, sound advice.

All foods fit into a healthy diet when the basic principles of balance and moderation are applied. A balanced daily diet is one that includes food from the five food groups. It is one in which portion sizes are proper and overindulging is avoided. Your daughter should be exposed to a variety of foods to help her appreciate different tastes and to avoid developing a habit of eating a few specific foods. Healthy eating also includes more than just what's on the table. Children should be allowed to eat in a stress-free environment, where manners are taught and used and where discussion is part of the social interaction of dining.[4]

> "Is it always inappropriate to give a child a cookie? No. But it's not always appropriate either . . . The parent has the responsibility to provide a variety of selections so that a sweet treat is just one of many foods offered in a day. In my opinion, never letting a kid have a sweet invests those foods with too much significance, which can cause problems later on."
>
> —Susan L. Johnson, of the Center for Human
> Nutrition at the University of Colorado

You may worry that purchasing low-fat foods will harm your child; that she needs plenty of fat in her diet. Children do need some fat. But they are getting far too much. Dietary guidelines recommend that anyone over the age of two get no more than 30 percent of their calories from fat. Sensible, low-fat diets will lower your daughter's cholesterol and reduce her risk of obesity without stunting growth.

Fruits and Vegetables

Most grade school children today learn about fruits and vegetables alongside their ABCs. Now, that's progress! So important are fruits and vegetables that they are now considered the "cornerstone" of a healthy diet. But there is evidence that we're a long way toward meeting the goal of five servings a day of fruits and vegetables. One survey found that, on average, children ate 4.7 servings of fruits and vegetables *a week*—which equals about half a serving a day.[5] And some of the servings of fruit consisted of fruit juice, which lacks fiber, a key component of fruit.

Given the emphasis on fruits and vegetables, you may be interested in providing vegetarian meals to your family. Questions have lingered, however, about whether a strict vegetarian diet is healthy for children. Your child can eat vegetarian as long as you oversee the diet carefully and plan meals with some precision. "Planning is the key," says Tammy Baker, an ADA spokesperson. "Any time you're excluding food groups, you have to be more careful to make sure you're still getting all the nutrients you need."[6] You need to watch for a few potential problems when going vegetarian. For one, the diets tend to be high on fiber, so children can fill up without getting all the calories for energy that they need. Nuts, seeds, dried fruits, and soy products can provide concentrated sources of calories. In addition, make sure your child's protein needs are being met through eating legumes, soy products, nuts, dairy products, and eggs. Other nutrients to watch for include calcium, vitamin D, iron, vitamin B_{12}, and zinc.

Breakfast Is a Must

A forgotten component of the healthy diet is breakfast. While it sounds trite, breakfast is still considered the most important meal of the day, particularly for children. Many children, however, do not eat a healthy breakfast or skip the meal entirely. Don't allow your daughter this freedom. Kids who eat a good breakfast learn better, are more alert, attentive, and healthier and are more likely to participate in activities such as sports.[7] Children who do not eat a good breakfast are more likely to be irritable, tired, have headaches or dizziness, suffer from more infections and colds, are less able to concentrate, miss more school days, and do poorer on standardized tests.[8] Students who skip breakfast can go up to sixteen hours (between the previous evening's snack and lunchtime) without nutrients. That leads to a mid-morning

Fruit and Vegetable Intake Falls Short

Well under 20% of kids eat at least five servings of fruits or vegetables a day. Fewer girls comply with the recommendation.

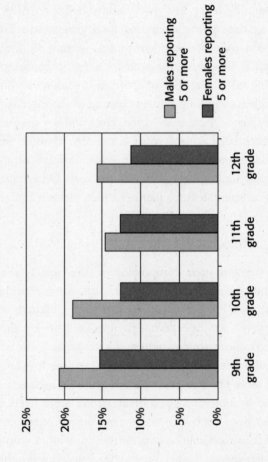

Males reporting 5 or more

Females reporting 5 or more

Source: Youth Risk Behavior Survey, MMRW 44(551) 1-55, 1995.

energy slump that can affect school performance. If it's hard to get breakfast together in the morning, enroll your child in her school's breakfast program if one is offered.

What Do Healthy Eating Habits Look Like?

While you are responsible for what is served, your daughter is responsible for what and how much she eats. Cajoling or forcing her to eat more or less of a food can contribute to disordered eating or anxiety about food. Donald, who has been a foster parent to dozens of girls, many with sad pasts and lingering emotional problems, has seen the power children can wield with their forks. "What is one thing a child can control? She can control what she eats," he says. "I talk to my daughters about eating well so they are healthy. And we have sit-down meals with fresh salads and vegetables. We focus on education and skill-building so the girl will succeed wherever she is."

Breakfast Burrito: This is an example of how to get good nutrition into your daughter's breakfast and impress her at the same time!

Ingredients

1 flour tortilla, heated
1 egg, scrambled
1 tablespoon salsa
1 tablespoon grated cheese

Lay the warm tortilla on a plate. Spread the cooked egg in the middle of the tortilla. Spoon the salsa on top of the egg and sprinkle with cheese. Fold one side of the tortilla over the egg, then roll up.

Source: American Dietetic Association.

Parents who impose strict mealtime rules on their children increase the risk that their children will develop unhealthy eating habits.[9] "Some children learn from controlling parents that their sense of hunger and fullness is irrelevant. When feeding turns into struggle for control, it makes it hard for children to develop self-control," says Susan Johnson, a nutrition expert at the University of Colorado Health Science Center.[10] Mothers tend to more closely control their daughter's eating habits than their son's. This type of pressure can result in a girl's preoccupation with thinness and dieting.

How to Set the Right Tone at Mealtimes

- Schedule meals and snacks.
- Eliminate interference. For example, turn off the TV at mealtime.
- Create a pleasant atmosphere for eating.
- Sit down and eat with your children. You can't be a role model if you're not there.
- Practice good table manners. Emphasize what children do right with compliments rather than criticism.
- Eat the same food the children eat. (If, for some reason, you cannot, explain why.)
- Prepare and serve a variety of foods that look and taste good.
- Be aware of portion sizes. Give children small portions and tell them they can have more if they want.
- No one needs to finish everything on her plate. Allow children to choose what and how much to eat. Respect individual taste preferences. Do not restrict favorite foods.
- Place no special merit on dessert. Dessert should not be a reward for eating "what's good for you."

Source: American Dietetic Association.

Patterns in Young Children

Children can begin to understand the properties of healthy eating but they may harbor some misconceptions. For example, many younger kids feel that their favorite foods are not good for them or believe foods that are healthy do not taste good.[11] Children should learn that all foods are fine in balance. Many young children are picky eaters and need to try a new food eight to ten times before accepting it.[12] If you have a picky eater, keep offering various foods while vowing to keep mealtime relaxed. Kelly is only nine, but her mother, Michelle, worries every day over her daughter's diet. "Kelly has always been a very picky eater," she says. "As of now she eats only pasta, cereal, cheese, bread, peanut butter, and dairy. No meat or vegetables and very little fruit. I do make sure she takes a multivitamin every day. I am afraid of making an issue out of her eating habits because I think it could create huge problems down the road."

Patterns in Preteens

Today, preteens often begin to adopt the poor diets that are typically not anticipated until the teen years. Few preteens will eat fruits or vegetables. Milk consumption declines and fondness for soda and sports drinks soars. More children today eat away from home than ever before.[13] Kids ages six through nineteen get about 25 percent of their food from places outside the home, such as restaurants and school food programs.[14] Kids are also eating more snack foods (such as crackers and cookies) and more high-fat convenience foods, such as TV dinners.

Ideas for Healthy Snacks

- Fresh or canned vegetables
- Fresh fruit
- Dried fruit, nuts, or sunflower seeds
- Breads or crackers made with whole grains served with fruit spreads or fat-free cheese
- Air-popped popcorn
- Low-fat or fat-free cookies
- Dry cereals served with low-fat or nonfat milk
- Frozen desserts such as nonfat or low-fat ice cream, frozen yogurt, Popsicles, and frozen fruit-juice bars

Source: National Institutes of Health.

Patterns in Adolescence

Adolescents typically eat at least one snack a day.[15] Snacks are okay to meet a teenager's energy needs, but problems can occur when the selection is always non-nutritious. Busy teens are also big purveyors of fast foods, vending-machine food, and convenience-store food. Because of teenagers' busy schedules away from home, it may become hard for you to have a lot of input into your daughter's diet. Moreover, part of being a teenager is expressing one's own identity, and that goes for food as well as clothes and music. Teens might even see junk food as a mild form of rebellion against the healthy family fare.[16] Or they take advantage of parents' busy schedules to indulge in non-nutritious choices. "I sometimes skip meals because I have homework," says Callie, fifteen. "Sometimes, my parents don't cook dinner. Then I eat junk food." As children near adulthood, fewer get even two-thirds of the daily recommendations for vitamins and minerals. For most teens, nutrition is simply not a priority. In an eye-opening survey of adolescents' perceptions of how much their peers cared about various health-related behaviors, "eating healthy food" was the *least valued* behavior.[18] And, controlling weight was the most highly valued behavior among eleven different behaviors, such as not using drugs and wearing seat belts.

Yes, it's tough getting a teenager to eat healthily. But if you don't at least remind your children of the importance of a healthy diet, teens will surely do little of their own accord. Helping your child eat healthy may also mean talking to others—especially school boards. Too many schools are overflowing with vending machines containing unhealthy food choices.

Other Tips to Grow a Nutrition-Conscious Girl

One of the great frustrations for all Americans is the conflicting reports about what is good for you and what isn't. Julie, the mother of two girls, thinks about this dilemma often. "I worry that there will be new research that says, 'By the way, you should have been feeding your kids more of (fill in the blank). So now your kids are at risk for (fill in the blank).' Oh well, I guess it doesn't pay to worry too much!" Julie's frustration is understandable. It seems that one week margarine is good and butter is bad, and the next week apple juice is bad and butter is good. And then eggs are bad and juice is good, and so on. Try not to worry about specific foods or nutrients (unless it is clear that your child has a specific deficiency, such as an iron deficiency). Instead, concentrate on providing a varied, healthy diet.

Many parents know about the Food Pyramid but don't use it to plan their meals. The Food Pyramid is simple to use, but is not really based on simple information. Foods are sorted into groups based on key nutrients representing more than forty nutrients needed by the body. Food can and should be eaten from each group (that is, one food group does not replace another). However, the recommended number of servings from each food

Kids Make Many Food Decisions

Many teens are involved in activities and decisions that affect their nutrition. The chart shows the percentage of teens who participated in these activities in an average week.

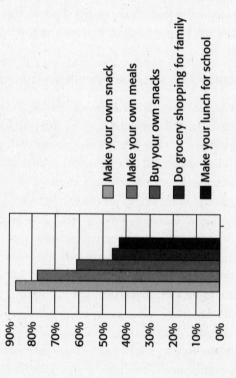

- Make your own snack
- Make your own meals
- Buy your own snacks
- Do grocery shopping for family
- Make your lunch for school

Source: National Dairy Council.

group will vary. It's not necessary to eat the exact number of recommended servings each day. Instead, aim for balance by averaging the proper number of servings over a week or two.

Other strategies for healthy eating include:

- Salt intake is linked to an increase in hypertension. Because of this, teach your teenager that excessive salt intake should be avoided. This is an important message considering that many favorite teen foods, such as potato chips, tortilla chips, popcorn, etc., are high in sodium. Send a message by leaving the salt shaker off the table.
- Lower fat intake further by choosing 1 percent or skim milk, low-fat yogurt, low-fat cheese, and very lean cuts of meat (such as 7 percent fat ground beef).
- Set regular mealtimes to help regulate appetite and establish patterns. A meal schedule also discourages overeating and snacking. Time snacks so that they are not close to a meal. Girls who fail to adjust what they eat in response to their pre-meal snack have the greatest amount of body fat.
- In the frantic pace of modern society, it's so tempting to resort to fast food for quick meals. Fast food is okay in moderation. But beware of the consequences if you find yourself eyeing the drive-thru sign night after night. Almost half of the calories in fast food come from fat.
- If there is one complaint heard over and over in the field of child and adolescent health it is the double whammy that children today experience by watching too much TV (instead of exercising) and being exposed to a flood of advertisements touting high-calorie, high-fat foods. One way you can deal with this is to strictly limit TV time. As for the advertisements, it's nearly impossible for children to avoid them. Advertisements are everywhere; not just on TV. You can help educate your child about TV food ads, however. Ask your child to describe how she thinks the manufacturer is trying to sell a

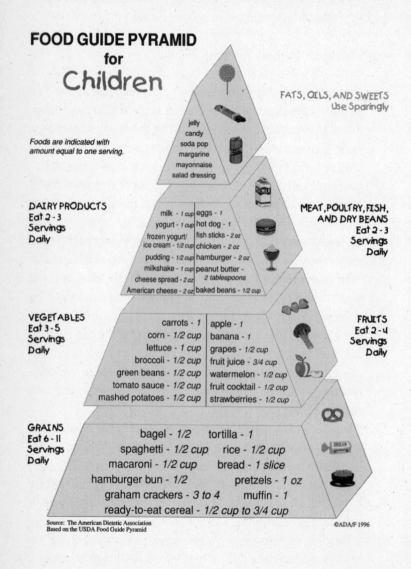

FOOD GUIDE PYRAMID
for
Children

Foods are indicated with amount equal to one serving.

FATS, OILS, AND SWEETS
Use Sparingly

jelly
candy
soda pop
margarine
mayonnaise
salad dressing

DAIRY PRODUCTS
Eat 2 - 3
Servings
Daily

milk - *1 cup*
yogurt - *1 cup*
frozen yogurt/ ice cream - *1/2 cup*
pudding - *1/2 cup*
milkshake - *1 cup*
cheese spread - *2 oz*
American cheese - *2 oz*

eggs - *1*
hot dog - *1*
fish sticks - *2 oz*
chicken - *2 oz*
hamburger - *2 oz*
peanut butter - *2 tablespoons*
baked beans - *1/2 cup*

MEAT, POULTRY, FISH, AND DRY BEANS
Eat 2 - 3
Servings
Daily

VEGETABLES
Eat 3 - 5
Servings
Daily

carrots - *1*
corn - *1/2 cup*
lettuce - *1 cup*
broccoli - *1/2 cup*
green beans - *1/2 cup*
tomato sauce - *1/2 cup*
mashed potatoes - *1/2 cup*

apple - *1*
banana - *1*
grapes - *1/2 cup*
fruit juice - *3/4 cup*
watermelon - *1/2 cup*
fruit cocktail - *1/2 cup*
strawberries - *1/2 cup*

FRUITS
Eat 2 - 4
Servings
Daily

GRAINS
Eat 6 - 11
Servings
Daily

bagel - *1/2*   tortilla - *1*
spaghetti - *1/2 cup*   rice - *1/2 cup*
macaroni - *1/2 cup*   bread - *1 slice*
hamburger bun - *1/2*
graham crackers - *3 to 4*   pretzels - *1 oz*
muffin - *1*
ready-to-eat cereal - *1/2 cup to 3/4 cup*

Source: The American Dietetic Association
Based on the USDA Food Guide Pyramid

©ADA/F 1996

particular food product. Ask if the commercial makes your child want the product more and whether the manufacturer is suggesting that eating the product will make a kid feel stronger, smarter, more popular, etc. Ask your child if she believes what the ad says. Point out that props and characters in the ad can make the food seem more appealing than it really is. Children should not be exploited in the pursuit of selling food. If you believe a food ad is out of bounds, complain to: Children's Advertising Review Unit, Council of Better Business Bureaus, 845 Third Avenue, New York, NY 10022.

A Look at Some Key Nutrients

Fiber: This is an important nutrient to promote normal bowel function in children and for disease prevention, such as gastrointestinal disorders, high cholesterol, and diabetes. A high-fiber diet helps prevent obesity. Follow this rule of thumb for

---

Parents' Tips for Getting Girls to Eat Smart

- "I rarely have junk food in the house in order to encourage snacking on healthy foods."
- "I read her a joke the other day. 'If you are what you eat, you're fast, cheap, and easy.' We just keeping working on nutrition."
- "I try constantly to point out nutritious foods and what vitamins do."
- "I never talk about diets or weight."
- "I have my daughter come home from school for lunch."
- "We emphasize vegetables and fruit, but we don't ban sweets."
- "We have sit-down meals with good foods—fresh salads and vegetables."
- "I always vary what I cook for dinner."
- "We talk to them about the importance of three balanced meals. They also always eat breakfast."

fiber intake in children older than two years of age: Dietary fiber intake should be equal to or greater than a child's age plus 5 grams a day.[19] For example, a ten-year-old girl should consume at least 15 grams a day.

High-Fiber Foods that Are Common in Children's Diets

Food	Serving size	Approx. grams of dietary fiber
Beans	1 c. baked	13
Chili with beans	1 c.	7
Almonds	2 oz. dry roasted	7
Peanuts	2 oz. dry roasted	4
Peanut butter	2 Tbsp.	2
Cereal	1 c.	(best choices have 3 g per cup)
Whole wheat bread	2 slices	4
Broccoli	½. c.	2
Corn	½ c.	3
Popcorn	2 c. popped	2
Potato	1 medium baked	2 (3.5 with skin)
Sweet potato	1 medium	3 (with skin)
Carrot	1 medium (raw)	3
Strawberries	1 c.	4
Pear	1 medium	4
Banana	1 large	3
Blueberries	1 c.	3
Apple	1 medium	3
Apricots	10 dried halves	3
Kiwi	1 large	3
Applesauce	½ c.	2

Source: "Importance of Dietary Fiber in Childhood," Christine L. Williams, *Journal of the ADA*, 1995.

Iron: It's not uncommon for girls to become low in iron. Be aware if your daughter's iron count is low, even if it is not so low that it qualifies as anemia. An estimated 25 percent of adolescent girls in the United States are iron deficient. The recommended daily intake of iron is 15 mg, but studies show that teen girls often get only 12 to 13 mg. Iron deficiency in infancy and childhood has been shown to cause changes in learning and behavior. The lack of iron can alter neurotransmitters, energy production, brain iron levels, protein production, and brain wave activity. One study found that teenage girls with iron deficiency who took iron supplements performed better on verbal learning tests than similar girls who did not take the supplements. Teen girls should be regularly tested for the iron levels in their blood because menstruation and rapid growth cause the body to need more iron. While most children are routinely monitored for anemia with a test that measures hemoglobin or hemocrit levels, an iron deficiency that doesn't meet the level of anemia will usually not be detected unless a girl receives a serum ferritin iron test. Many health experts believe that girls should be given this test and monitored for iron deficiency from childhood through the teen years.

Zinc: This is an important mineral to children, particularly during adolescence. During periods of rapid growth, zinc requirements increase from 10 to 15 mg per day. Zinc is found in abundance in fish, poultry, meat, peas, beans, and some cereals. Ideally, girls should get zinc and iron in similar amounts.

Folic acid: While this nutrient has received much attention as crucial to women at the time they become pregnant, the role is also important to children because it may have some cancer-fighting properties. However, studies show that females twelve to nineteen often fall short of the recommended intake of 400 ug per day. Folic acid is found in dark green, leafy vegetables, melons, and other fruits and whole grains. Girls who attempt to eat five servings a day of fruits and vegetables would meet this goal.

Calcium: This nutrient is so important to girls that a special chapter is devoted to it. See chapter 1.

Questions to Ask Your Doctor

- What can I do to encourage my child to eat more fruits and vegetables?
- How often is it okay to eat at fast-food restaurants?
- What kinds of snacks should I offer to my child?
- How do I encourage my daughter to try new foods without turning dinnertime into a battleground?
- My teenager drinks a lot of soda. Is that okay?
- When was the last time my daughter's iron was checked in a blood test?
- What would be the best type of supplement to give my daughter, given her diet?

Some of the Nutrients Represented by Each Food Group

Food Group	Key Nutrients
Bread, cereal, rice, pasta	Carbohydrates, B vitamins, some fiber
Vegetable	Vitamins A & C, folic acid, fiber
Fruit	Vitamins A & C, folic acid, fiber
Milk, yogurt, cheese	Calcium, riboflavin, protein
Meat, poultry, fish, beans, eggs, nuts	Protein, iron, zinc, fiber (in beans and nuts)
Fats, oils, sweets	Essential fatty acids, vitamin E, carbohydrates (from sweets)

Resources

- To order the brochure for kids ages nine to fifteen entitled *10 Tips to Healthy Eating and Physical Activity For You*, contact the American Dietetic Association, 800-366-1655.
- Teenagers who are vegetarians might enjoy a book written especially for them that explains how to adopt a healthy vegetarian diet. It also includes recipes. *Vegetables Rock: A Complete Guide for Teenage Vegetarians*, by Stephanie Pierson (Bantam, 1999).
- Tufts University operates a wonderful nutrition web site called the Nutrition Navigator at www.navigator.tufts.edu.
- Another site for kids is the Dole 5-A-Day home page at www.dole5aday.com.
- *American Academy of Pediatrics Guide to Your Child's Nutrition*, by Dr. William H. Dietz and Dr. Loraine Stern (Villard, 1998).
- *Great Girl Food: Easy Eats and Tempting Treats for Girls to Make*, American Girl Library, Pleasant, Co.
- The International Food and Information Council has lots of good information for parents at http://ificinfo.health.org.
- The Kids Food Cyber Club, a web site from the Connecticut Association for Human Services and Kaiser Permanente, helps make nutrition fun. You can find it at www.kidsfood.org.
- The Nemours Foundation Center for Children's Health Media sponsors a terrific web site for kids on nutrition. Kids can learn about food labels, healthy foods, and recipes they can make. There is also information for parents. Visit www.kidshealth.org.

CHAPTER 8

Eating Disorders: The Thin Line Between Normal and Dangerous

Aᴌᴌ ᴍʏ ʟɪꜰᴇ I had a strange relationship with food," says Caroline, now nineteen. "It hit high gear in high school, and I dabbled in anorexia before I became a full-fledged bulimic, mostly with laxatives. My body was always something I loathed. I cannot express how horrible my life was. High school was bad enough without this rearing its ugly head every day. Every single night of bingeing and purging was a battle—a battle I tried desperately to win but couldn't, of course. My parents didn't understand, even though my mother pressured me a lot to be the best at everything, which included looking good. At one time in my life she said if I gained five pounds, I owed her money. Of course, I had my dramatic hospital stays and therapy sessions, and when I went to college it all really blew up in my face. My life became so meaningless. I wanted the meaning back so badly. So, I slowly stopped. I started going to class and going out. My parents learned about bulimia and the few close friends I have supported me. I still have negative feelings about my body. Throughout this whole process my body has changed in so many ways that it's been hard to control myself so many times. Sometimes, I relapse, and I yearn for the day I can eat a 'normal,' medium-sized, healthy meal without thinking too much about it. Is that too much to ask?"

Eating disorders are not new diseases. Anorexia was described as early as 1694. But surely no other era has seen such a high prevalence of eating disorders than among American girls at the end of the twentieth century. It's not hard to think of several famous women who have succumbed to the disorder. For example, singer Karen Carpenter, gymnast Christy Heinrich, and Princess Diana, all now dead, the first two having died from complications related to eating disorders. There are many other, anonymous girls, like Caroline who remind us that eating disorders are in every school, every neighborhood.

Victims of eating disorders are usually female (90 percent of cases), white (95 percent of cases), and teenagers (75 percent of cases) when first diagnosed.[1] According to the National Institute of Mental Health, cases of anorexia and bulimia have doubled over the past decade. In recent years, more cases have been seen in African-American and Asian girls growing up in Western cultures where thinness is valued.[2] While teenagers are the most likely to be diagnosed with eating disorders, the problems are appearing with greater frequency among children from ages nine to twelve. Early diagnosis among preteens is essential because younger girls with eating disorders have the worst prognosis. Unfortunately, very few parents or even pediatricians think about the possibility of disordered eating in children that young and, therefore, often fail to recognize a problem before it is too late.

"I thought about drugs, sex, pregnancy, violence in schools, car safety—but never eating disorders. I did not realize the prevalence in my own community, never mind in my own household," says Sheryl, whose daughter, Amy, was on the cusp of early adolescence when Sheryl noticed that her daughter was thinner, looked tired, and acted withdrawn. "But, in all actuality, I did not know she had an eating disorder until she came and told me she thought she had a problem. Looking back, she always had gum in her mouth. She did binge, and she was more difficult than usual. Because she is a vegetarian, she tended to eat more frequently and in somewhat larger quantities than the rest of us. But what I did not realize was then she would go and eliminate all the food."

Some experts object to the term "eating disorder" because it implies that the problem has to do with learning to eat normally again, says nutritionist Frances M. Berg, editor and publisher of the *Healthy Weight Journal* and author of *Afraid to Eat*. It's not so simple as just learning how to eat normally again. Eating disorders include not only problems with food and eating, Berg explains, but with emotions and relationships.

Eating disorders are psychiatric illnesses. These disorders are often very difficult for outsiders to understand. Food, for most of us, is a source of pleasure or simple sustenance. Obsessions over food and weight in young women are even more perplexing. How can a razor-thin teenager with bones jutting against her skin look in a mirror and see a fat girl? Increasingly, researchers are suggesting that eating disorders involve serious alterations of brain chemistry. New research may lead to better treatments that address imbalances in neurochemical circuits in the brain.

Several other theories focus on a combination of personality characteristics and family dynamics. Sexual or physical abuse is thought to be a major risk factor for eating disorders.[3] Another study suggested that girls with chronic illnesses, such as asthma, diabetes, seizure disorders, and attention deficit disorder are more likely to be dissatisfied with their bodies and develop eating disorders.[4] And, many experts wonder whether the mere prevalence with dieting is, in and of itself, enough to trigger some cases of eating disorders. According to one study, girls who dieted were eight times more likely to develop eating disorders than girls who did not diet.[5]

Chelsea is a teenager who has struggled with bulimia and anorexia since age twelve. It all started, she says, with an obsession over her body. "I was trying to be beautiful and I thought the thinner I was, the more beautiful I would be. I wanted to impress guys and I thought the thinner I was, the more guys I would attract. I looked at those glamour magazines and I thought 'that's the way I'm supposed to look.' " Marla, sixteen, describes her descent into bulimia this way: "I would diet and exercise every day until I dropped. I would look at my sister, who is large, and tell myself I am not going to be like her. I think society plays a part in how girls think they should be thin and beautiful."

But there is no one simple explanation to explain the prevalence of eating disorders.

> "Families of eating disordered youth are in a difficult situation. They see their child behaving in destructive ways and feel helpless and frustrated. They may try to gain control over what and how much the teenager chooses to eat. Some police washrooms and search through drawers for pills and laxative. Moms and dads struggle with both the child's problem eating and their own concerns over injury to growth and development. The eating disorder may take over and dominate family life."
>
> —Frances M. Berg, author of *Children and Teens Afraid to Eat*: *Helping Youth in Today's Weight-Obsessed World*. Revised edition, 2000.

What Is Anorexia?

Anorexia nervosa is used to describe people who avoid putting on weight or try to lose weight by severe food restrictions. Experts usually use the following criteria to diagnose the disorder:[6]

- A refusal to maintain body weight at or above 85 percent of what is normal based on age and height
- An intense fear of gaining weight or getting fat
- An inability to perceive one's body weight or shape correctly and denial of the seriousness of the current low body weight
- In girls who have already reached puberty, the absence of at least three consecutive menstrual cycles

Other signs of anorexia:

- Developing rituals around eating, such as cutting food into tiny pieces
- Denying hunger
- Exercising excessively
- Eating only low- or nonfat food
- A self-image of being fat when this is not true
- Hiding feelings

Anorexia is a disorder that is most common in societies like ours, where thinness is desired as the ultimate beauty trait. The disorder usually surfaces between the ages of thirteen and twenty.[7] Researchers estimate that about one out of every 100 girls will develop anorexia.[8] Anorectics will avoid eating or will develop strange habits, such as cutting up their food into tiny pieces or eating only certain foods. As many as 75 percent of anorectics exercise to burn off calories.[9]

No one really knows what causes anorexia or any eating disorder. Genetics may play a role because the disorder does run in families. Rates also appear higher in families that have other types of mental illnesses, such as depression or obsessive-compulsive disorder or anxiety. Many anorexics are also diagnosed with one of these illnesses. Researchers also think that a girl's environment contributes to the disease. Unhealthy eating practices, negative mealtime atmosphere, and being forced to eat are factors that are typically seen among anorexics. Family dysfunction may contribute to the disease. Overly rigid or controlling parents are sometimes thought to contribute to the emergence of the disorder. As Wisconsin therapist Ellyn Satter describes it: "Eating is a sensitive barometer of emotional state and parent-child interaction."[10] Sheryl, Amy's mother, sees several trends in her daughter's life that all flowed into an eating disorder. "When Amy was in middle school, she was teased and tormented because she was chubby. This left her with a horrible self-image and self-esteem. Contributing to the problem was a lack of attention from her father. This led Amy to feel inadequate, not athletically inclined (like her brothers were), and, in general, a loser. She also took ballet for many years and enjoyed it very much. But she compared herself to other dancers in her classes who had the perfect dancers' bodies."

Some researchers suggest that girls develop eating disorders as a way to exercise control in their otherwise chaotic lives. Girls with anorexia are also prone to be perfectionists who are eager to please others and meet their expectations. These girls may use eating as a way to address other problems in their lives. For example, says Satter, they believe that they'll be loved better by their parents if they're thinner. Or they won't think about their troubles in school so much if they focus intensely on their diets. Crystal, now seventeen, was so competitive that even her eating disorder became a battle of winners and losers. "It's become more like addictive behavior," she says. "In order to 'win' I need to be the thinnest person in the world and the best at my eating disorder."

> "An eating disorder of childhood is the misuse of feeding in an attempt to solve or camouflage family problems . . . that seem otherwise insoluble. The childhood eating disorder might take the form of failure to thrive, obesity, excessive finickiness, or most commonly, vehement and protracted struggles between a parent and child about eating."
>
> —Ellyn Satter, eating disorders specialist

Only a qualified mental health professional can diagnose anorexia. Your pediatrician can refer you to such a specialist. If detected early, the chances of recovery are much better. But, overall, recovery is difficult to attain. For many girls, the disease is a chronic condition that requires constant therapy and dedication to recovery. Even an initial phase of treatment can last up to two years. There are many types of therapy, but most focus on a combination of psychotherapy and medication. About 40 percent of all anorectics will have a bulimic phase during the course of their treatment or recovery.[11] Often, hospitalization is necessary to restore a girl's weight to a functional level.

It is imperative that families make every effort and exhaust all options to find effective treatments for their daughters. The disease, if allowed to persist, can cause serious medical complications. Anorectics typically have abnormal thyroid function as well as respiratory and blood pressure rates. They lose calcium in their bones, develop anemia and swollen joints, and abnormal heart rhythms. Even their brains can shrink. About 5 percent to 18 percent of anorectics eventually die of starvation or cardiac arrest.[12] Even with the best possible therapy, it's not easy for families to watch a child struggle with an eating disorder. The family cannot make the child adopt healthy eating patterns. The child herself has to respond to treatment with some voluntary effort. "She wouldn't eat anything but lettuce and salad. And I noticed her rapid weight loss," says Alicia, the mother of a girl who is severely ill with anorexia and bulimia. "At the very first sign, parents need to get help. Get into counseling. Don't let it go on. I had to sit by and watch someone I love very much dying. And I couldn't do anything about it."

What Is Bulimia?

Bulimia is actually more common than anorexia; an estimated 2 percent to 3 percent of adolescent girls suffer from bulimia.[13] Symptoms of bulimia or partial bulimia have been reported in as many as 40 percent of college women.[14] Bulimia is seen in girls who are usually of normal weight or perhaps slightly overweight. It is thought that purging (by vomiting or using lax-

---

Factors that May Contribute to Eating Disorders

- Being female, especially if obese or over-concerned with thinness, in a culture where thinness is highly valued.
- Being perfectionistic and eager to please others, but not able to consider one's own needs. Candace, a teenager with an eating disorder, found that her tendency to want to please others was a factor in her illness. "It had a lot to do with the perfect image. I tried to please my parents at all costs. When my parents found out about it, they said I did it for attention."
- Having difficulty communicating negative emotions such as anger, sadness, or fear.
- Having difficulty resolving conflict.
- Having low self-esteem.

Source: Pediatrics in Review.

atives) provides relief after bingeing. Bulimics are typically impulsive and may have other personality disturbances. [15] To diagnose the disorder, these criteria are often cited:[16]

- Recurrent episodes of binge eating at least twice a week for three months
- Recurrent purging behavior to prevent weight gain, including vomiting, misuse of laxatives, diuretics, enemas, fasting, or exercise
- Attitude that places too much emphasis on weight or shape

Other signs of bulimia:[17]

- Making excuses to use the rest room after meals
- Unusual swelling around the jaw
- Frequent eating of a large amount of high-calorie food but no weight gain.

Bulimia may have causes that are rooted in brain chemicals called neurotransmitters. The chemicals serotonin and norepinephrine play a role in depression and may also lead to bulimia. Bulimia often runs in families. Families with high rates of substance abuse and mental disorders tend to have higher rates of bulimia as well.

Bulimia is a disorder that should be treated with alarm. Even occasional vomiting episodes should not be tolerated as normal or part of "a stage." A ruptured stomach or esophagus can occur with bulimia. The disorder also causes great stress on the heart and can produce serious electrolyte imbalances that can lead to heart failure. Cardiac arrhythmias are common in bulimics. The vomiting can also wear down the enamel on teeth.

Bulimics are typically easier to spot and may not even try to hide the disorder. Thus, getting a girl into treatment is usually a little easier than with anorectics. Bulimics are usually treated with a combination of therapies that include counseling and medication. The newer antidepressants, called selective serotonin reuptake inhibitors, have shown to be helpful to some bulimics.

What Is Binge Eating?

Binge eating has only recently been included in the family of eating disorders. Binge eaters overeat, as do many bulimics. But while bulimics purge themselves of food, binge eaters do not attempt to rid themselves of the extra calories. The disorder is usually described this way:

- Recurrent episodes of overeating
- A feeling of losing control when eating and eating to excess

Other signs of binge eating disorder:

- Frequently eats a large amount of food that is more than most people would eat
- Eats rapidly
- Eats alone
- Eats to the point of being uncomfortable

About 30 percent of people who enter weight-control programs are binge eaters (or about 2 percent of the general population).[18] Most binge eaters are obese and have battled their weight for a long time. Oftentimes, binge eaters are also diagnosed with depression. Binge eaters suffer the same risks as obese people, such as higher rates of heart disease, cancer, diabetes, hypertension, and gallbladder disease. The treatment is much like that for bulimia; a combination of medication and therapy with an emphasis on proper nutrition and exercise.

Treatment for Eating Disorders

"It's important for both parents and teens to know as much as they can about eating disorders and what to do if their child or best friend is showing signs of the condition."

—Carol Noel, author of *Get It? Got It? Good!*
A Guide for Teenagers

"To think that your child is unhappy and not be able to fix it is hard to swallow. This is something that she has to do on her own. I can only support her. I can't do it for her. I can't buy her things to compensate for her misery, can't force her to eat, and can't follow her into the bathroom after every meal. As a parent, we have a desire to fix all problems. But this one cannot be fixed by me alone. This is a group effort with professionals such as psychiatrists, nutritionists, pediatricians, guidance counselors, and eating disorder specialists, as well as family support and her strong will to be better," says Sheryl, of Amy, who is now in high school and continues to have eating problems.

In 1995, medical experts released the first guidelines for treating adolescents with eating disorders.[19] In this report, experts advised that any teenager who engages in potentially unhealthy weight-control practices or who seem obsessed with food, weight, body shape, or exercise, should be evaluated for a possible eating disorder. "In adults, weight loss has been the standard hallmark for diagnosing eating disorders. In adolescents, however, a more revealing clue may be the failure to gain or maintain an age-appropriate weight," said the authors of the report.

It's important for families with this problem to obtain the guidelines. (See Resources for information.) Teens with eating disorders cannot be treated in the same way that adults with eating disorders are treated. Families also need to think about whether their health insurance policies cover the treatment of eating disorders. Many policies do not. While we, as parents, never want to believe that something so horrible could befall our daughters, it would be prudent to know if your insurance policy covers this treatment. Families in which there is a history of eating disorders or mental illnesses should be especially attuned to insurance coverage. And, families in which girls have already shown signs of struggling with food issues should make sure they are covered. If the time comes when you need to obtain help for your daughter, you will be thankful that you have the insurance resources to obtain the best help available.

It may be very difficult to convince your daughter that she needs counseling for an eating problem. Jerrie, fifteen, is seriously ill with bulimia and sees a therapist twice a week, and a nutritionist and a physician once a week. But, she says: "I don't want to go. I'm not scared. I just hate being told what to do. I want to be perfect, and get better on my own."

A hallmark of the disease is denial. One study found that six out of ten high school girls with eating disorders or symptoms of disorders did not think they needed counseling for their behavior.[20] Girls may be particularly reluctant to think of the behavior as abnormal if they see so many of their friends engaged in similar disordered eating patterns. "I think a lot of young girls start to believe disordered eating is normal because they see their friends doing it," says Dinah Meyer, the author of a study on girls with eating disorders. "They minimize the behavior and say it's no big deal . . . It's important to intervene before their eating behaviors get worse. Just as parents are taught to look for drug use in their teens, they should be taught to look for eating disorder behaviors, too."

"It has been a long struggle. Anyone who wants this is stupid. You don't want this. It cost me a scholarship and I had no life. It hurts your family and friends, too."

—Elizabeth, sixteen, an anorectic

Lesser Versions of Eating Disorders

Besides the high numbers of girls with full-blown eating disorders, many more girls are thought to have milder versions of the disorders or partial disorders in which maybe only one or two symptoms are present. In fact, an estimated 5 percent to 10 percent of adolescents and young adult women are thought to have lesser versions of eating disorders.[21] The one central factor among these cases is that sometime around puberty, girls become excessively conscious of their weight and feel that they should start dieting.

Eating disorders are often triggered in girls who fear their physical maturation.[22] Among younger girls with eating disorders (prior to puberty) there may be a hidden desire to remain a child. Some girls may not understand that gaining weight and acquiring a fuller and rounder body is a normal part of puberty, not a sign she is getting "fat." Girls, far more than boys, are more likely to overestimate their body weight, And, according to one expert, this tendency to overestimate body weight is more prevalent in girls at age eleven.[23] Among older teenagers, the struggle for independence or control seems to be more strongly linked to eating disorders. Developing symptoms may be a way of acting out to assert autonomy. In girls approaching high school graduation, an eating disorder may signify an identity crisis and a fear of what the remainder of their life may hold.

> "I've seen students with advanced eating disorders seeking help only after they've finally fainted while exercising. Even then, it often takes an extended period for students with eating disorders to admit they have been eating practically nothing and exercising compulsively."
>
> —Kathy Hotelling, president of the Association of University and College Counseling Center Directors

How do parents know when they are seeing the early signs of disordered eating? This is not an easy task, say nutrition experts Lucy B. Adams and Mary-Ann B. Shafer. "It is often difficult to distinguish between a teen with 'normal' eating habits and one with an eating disorder.[24] Adolescent eating habits are typically characterized by meal skipping, snacking, food choices low in nutrient density, and frequent meals eaten away from home. In addition, as a normal part of adolescent development, adolescents may diet, or try food fads." They explain that eating disorders can be viewed as "a continuum from nondieters and simple experimenters or occasional dieters to the clinical extreme of bulimia nervosa and anorexia nervosa."

The major method of distinguishing between harmless food habits and a dangerous disorder lies in the frequency of the behavior (How often does your daughter go all day without eating?), the extent of food- or weight-related concerns (Is her worrying over her weight an excessive preoccupation or one of many complaints she has about herself or her life?), and the presence of medical symptoms (Has there been a sudden weight loss or have her periods stopped?).

Parents can help assess their daughter's risk of developing an eating disorder by taking an objective look at the family's nutrition, meals, eating habits, and general functioning. Girls who grow up in families where there is much discussion over dieting or where there is a history of obesity or eating disorders are at higher risk of developing a problem. Studies of girls with eating disorders show that many can pinpoint a stressful time in their lives when the disorder seemed to kick in, such as the parents' divorce, a move, or a death in the family. Moreover, parents need to examine a girl's activities. Girls involved in ballet, modeling, gymnastics, cheerleading, and other activities in which a slender body is highly prized are at higher risk. Finally, parents need to be aware that messages in the media that prize thinness are absorbed

Comparing the Behavior of Normal Adolescents with Eating Disordered Behavior

This chart shows how much normal teenager behavior can appear similar to eating disordered behavior. However, a few telltale signs of eating disorders, such as laxative and diet pill use, cannot be construed as normal adolescent behavior. (*Y* means yes, the behavior might be present, while *N* means no, the behavior isn't usually present.)

Feature	Normal teen	Bulimic	Anorexic
Binge eating episode	Y/N	Y	Y/N
Dissatisfaction with weight or shape	Y/N	Y	Y
Extreme fear of gaining weight	Y/N	Y	Y
Frequent meal skipping	Y	Y	Y
Frequent snacking	Y	Y	Y
Frequent vomiting or laxative use	N	Y	Y/N
Guilt after eating	Y/N	Y	Y
Poor coping with stressful life event	Y/N	Y/N	Y/N
Preoccupied with food	Y/N	Y	Y
Regular diet pill use	N	Y/N	Y/N
Restrictive dieting	Y/N	Y/N	Y
Uncomfortable eating with others	Y/N	Y	Y/N

Source: Lucy B. Adams and Mary-Ann B. Shafer, M.D., "Early Manifestations of Eating Disorders in Adolescents," *Journal of Clinical Nutrition*, Vol. 20, No. 6, 1988.

by our daughters without challenge—unless we, as parents, make a point of educating our daughters about the unnaturalness of those images and how they set unrealistic and harmful expectations for women. If you think your daughter shows signs of disordered eating, it's important to seek the consultation of your family physician or pediatrician and, perhaps, a registered dietitian or expert in eating disorders as well.

Warning Signs for Anorexia Nervosa

Eating and related behaviors

Caloric intake under 1000 calories a day
Calorie counting
Denial of hunger cues
Extreme physical activity
Fasting or restrictive dieting
Feels controlled by food
Food avoidances or hoarding
Food seen as good or bad
Frequent meal skipping
Frequent thoughts about food

Body image and body satisfaction

Body image disturbance
Fear of weight gain
Previously overweight
Thinness as valued goal
Weight goal less than 85 percent of expected weight

Health status

Amenorrhea for three or more months
Bloating and nausea

Cold intolerance

Constipation

Weight equal to or less than 85 percent of expected weight

Personal functioning

Delayed psychosexual development

Depressed mood

Individuation difficulties

Negative self-image

Perfectionistic

Poor coping with a life event

Recent withdrawal from friends

Environmental influences

Enmeshed or overinvolved family

Family history of obesity, eating disorder, or weight focus

Few close friends

High-achievement expectations

Participation in body-focused activity

Warning Signs for Bulimia Nervosa

Eating and related behaviors

Binge eating more than twice a week

Eating used as coping strategy

Fasting or restrictive dieting

Feels lack of control over eating

Frequent meal skipping

Frequent sweets, starches, cravings

Frequent thoughts about food

Guilt after eating

Secret eating

Purging behavior
Regular alcohol use
Wide variation in caloric intake

Body image and body satisfaction

Current or previous obesity
Fear of weight gain
Overconcern with weight shape
Thinness as valued goal
Unrealistic weight goal

Health status

Bloating, nausea, abdominal pain
Constipation
Frequent weight fluctuations
Irregular menstruation, such as less than twenty-one days or
    greater than forty-five days

Personal functioning

Depressed mood
Negative self-esteem
Perfectionistic
Poor coping with life event
Recent withdrawal from friends
Substance use, early sexual activity

Environmental influences

Chaotic or uninvolved family
Family history of obesity, eating disorder, weight, or fitness focus
High-achievement expectations
Participation in body-focused activity[25]

Tips to Prevent Eating Disorders

1. Discourage restrictive dieting, meal skipping, or fasting.
2. Provide information about the normal changes during puberty.
3. Correct misconceptions about nutrition, normal body weight, and healthy approaches to weight loss.
4. Carefully phrase any weight-related recommendations or comments. Remember these words from Tricia, fifteen, who has anorexia: "Do not tell girls that they look better. 'Cause when someone says I look better I go out and lose ten pounds."
5. Refer an adolescent who appears to have an eating problem to a physician and/or mental health professional skilled in working with eating disorder patients.[26]

Talk to your daughter about eating disorders, even if she shows no sign of having a problem with food. Let her know, up front, that they are among the most common and fatal of all adolescent health problems.

Questions to Ask Your Doctor

- My daughter has lost weight. Could this be a sign of a possible eating disorder?
- My daughter disappears into the bathroom for a long time after meals. Is this normal behavior?
- I believe my daughter has an eating disorder but she denies it. How should I go about having a health expert evaluate her if she's uncooperative?
- I think my daughter eats too much and too fast. How can I get her to alter her behavior?
- Can you refer me to a therapist who has a special expertise in eating disorders among girls?

- I want to talk to my daughter about preventing eating disorders, but isn't that putting ideas in her head?

Resources

- The National Association of Anorexia Nervosa and Associated Disorders, P.O. Box 7, Highland Park, IL 60035. Call 847-831-3438.
- The American Anorexia/Bulimia Association, Inc., 418 East Seventeenth Street, New York, NY 10021. Call 212-575-6200 or visit www.aabainc.org.
- *The Best Little Girl in the World*, by Steven Levenkron (Warner Books, 1979).
- *Children and Teens Afraid to Eat: Helping Youth in Today's Weight-Obsessed Culture,* revised edition, by Frances M. Berg (Healthy Weight Publishing Network, 2000). To order: 701-567-2646.

CHAPTER 9

Preventing Major Diseases: Now Is the Time

M Y GRANDMA died of diabetes," says Jessica, fifteen. "My mom, my sister, and me are all overweight. My dad is so worried about us getting diabetes. He put us all on a diet."

Jessica may think her father is overreacting. But, in fact, many of the major illnesses that eventually kill adults have their roots in childhood and adolescence. They are linked to major lifestyle habits, such as diet and exercise, that begin to take shape early in life.

Parents who are battling health problems that are strongly related to lifestyle habits—such as diabetes, heart disease, and hypertension—would be wise to consider whether their children are developing risk factors for the same illnesses. For example,

Tara and Reggie, who have two daughters, are both overweight. Tara, fifty-one, also has a heart condition and high blood pressure. Reggie is hypertensive. But Tara feels the deepest anxiety when she looks at her beloved girls, Corinne, fifteen, and Meggie, twelve. "Corinne and Meggie eat a lot of junk and love it. I must admit that we eat out too often. I guess I need to work on that. Corinne is very tall but still falls into the overweight charts. With Meggie, weight is not yet an issue. But we are all concerned about our weight. They know that I take pills for both heart and blood pressure and that they will probably have problems if they don't watch it now."

Tara and Reggie are right to be concerned. If they looked carefully at their pasts, they could probably identify factors in childhood that led to their own cardiovascular problems.

> "We now know that (heart disease) risk factors important in adulthood are just as crucial in children."
>
> —Dr. Claude Lenfant, former director of the
> National Heart, Lung and Blood Institute

It's difficult to consider serious diseases like heart disease and cancer affecting our daughters. But they are affecting many of our children. Right now. This very minute. The forces that cause many devastating diseases begin in childhood and progress slowly and silently until they emerge much later in life as full-blown, possibly fatal, illnesses. We need to recognize that disease is essentially the end point of a long process that begins quietly early in life. For example, Tara understands that her older daughter's weight problem and love of junk food are the underpinnings of future heart disease. And she is determined to step in and steer Corinne away from that possibility. What Tara and Reggie need to do is no mystery. Many of the fundamentals of good health that we've already discussed—nutrition, exercise, stress management—apply to the prevention of many deadly diseases. If we can urge our girls to embrace a few simple health values and practices, they will be well on their way to reducing the risk of some of the most common diseases of our time. That information should help them feel confident and in control of their future health. Misa has told her nine-year-old daughter, Tamar, that heart disease and obesity are prevalent in their family. But she can add this confident addendum: "I tell her that since we now eat healthy, the risk is much lower!"

Heart Disease

The disease that kills more women is the one that probably worries them least. And it is also probably the most preventable serious disease with its roots in childhood.

Heart disease kills more women than any other illness—far more than all forms of cancer combined. One in eight women will ultimately die of some form of heart disease.[1]

Yet, this disease of late life typically begins before age twenty, and is centered around three risk factors—high-density lipoprotein, low-density lipoprotein, and smoking. (HDL, or high-density lipoprotein, helps remove cholesterol from the arteries and high levels are good. LDL helps deposit cholesterol and high levels are bad. Smoking increases the risk of heart disease and aortic aneurysm, in which the main heart artery widens and can burst).

Many girls are already pushing the odds that they will develop heart disease. Almost 14 million girls ages nineteen and under have excessive serum cholesterol levels of 170 mg/dl or higher.[2] In children and teens, total cholesterol levels should be under 170 mg/dl. Obesity, which affects about one in five girls, is another ominous sign. Children who are overweight early in life have higher risks for heart disease. Children with fat bellies, in particular, are at greater risk.[3] Examining all the risks factors

---

Risk Factors for Heart Disease That Can Be Identified Early in Life:

- **Smoking**—Smokers have a two to six times higher risk of heart attack. Women smokers who use oral contraceptives are up to thirty-nine times more likely to have a heart attack and up to twenty-two times more likely to have a stroke compared to women who don't smoke or use birth control pills.
- **High blood pressure**—After age sixty-five, nearly sixty-eight percent of women are hypertensive.
- **Physical inactivity**—Nearly doubles the risk for heart disease.
- **Cholesterol**—Women with low HDL cholesterol and high levels of triglycerides are at greatest risk.
- **Family history**—Daughters of parents with heart disease are at higher risk.
- **Age**—Older than fifty-five or premature menopause without use of estrogen replacement therapy increases risk.
- **Race**—African-American women have greater risk of heart disease because they typically have higher average blood pressure levels.
- **Obesity**—Those 30 percent or more over ideal body weight are at greater risk.

Source: American Heart Association, 1993.

---

shows that children today, if not assisted in becoming healthier, will one day yield a generation of adults with soaring levels of heart disease. One study of 7,000 people ages six to twenty-four found risk factors in heart disease are prevalent in some children as young as age nine.[4]

"It is well documented that cardiovascular disease is the leading cause of death among women, accounting for nearly 500,000 deaths each year. Yet, heart disease continues to be treated as a problem of middle-aged men. We're setting out to change that. It's time we stopped just talking and made a monumental change in how we diagnose and treat women."

—Dr. Debra R. Judelson, former vice president
of the American Medical Women's
Association

It is also time we recognized that heart disease prevention for women begins in girlhood, and that we know how to dramatically reduce the odds of developing the disease through a low-fat diet, emphasis on fruits and vegetables in the diet, not smoking, sufficient exercise, and stress reduction. Practicing any one of these prevention principles will be helpful. But scientists were startled to find recently that the benefits can be compounded. The vast majority of all heart disease in women could be eradicated if women adhered to *all the guidelines* to lower heart disease. For example, women who don't smoke, get thirty minutes or more of daily exercise, eat a diet rich in fruits and vegetables, avoid saturated fat, are not overweight, and have less than one alcoholic drink per day cut their chances of developing heart disease by 82 percent.[5] That is far above the previous estimates that combining all the protective factors could cut the risk by 50 percent.

Still, this same study found that very few of the adult women surveyed actually followed this complete regimen. One possible explanation for this is that many adult women may have become sedentary or started smoking decades ago and now find it agonizingly hard to change their behavior. Once bad habits are established, they are difficult to change. Children, however, can easily learn heart-healthy behaviors. Girls in grades three to five, for example, have been shown to be very receptive to instruction about diets low in fat.[6] However, the effects of instruction fade over the middle and high school years if children don't receive reminders or repeated messages. Clarissa has already started to explain to her daughter, Denise, nine, how poor health habits cause disease. "I want her to know what triggers it and how important good eating habits and exercise are to combat disease."

Treating Hypertension and High Cholesterol Early in Life

Hypertension in your daughter should be taken very seriously. If the problem surfaces in childhood, the child is likely to remain hypertensive in adulthood unless a successful intervention is undertaken.[7] There is also strong evidence that a family history of hypertension is a significant risk factor for a child developing the disorder and can lead to emergence of higher-than-normal blood pressure readings in girls as young as age nine.[8]

In the past, doctors have disagreed about the accuracy of blood pressure readings in children. This is no longer the case, thanks to federal guidelines released in 1996. The new standards set by the National Heart, Lung and Blood Institute list blood pressure according to height percentiles for children up to the age of seventeen. This is important because body size is the most important determinant of blood pressure in youth, and children grow at varying rates, so adjustments must be made to interpret readings for each individual. With the new guidelines, very tall children who will naturally have higher blood pressure levels are less likely to be misdiagnosed and very short children with high blood pressure will not be overlooked.[9]

Children with elevated blood pressure should be treated with nondrug therapies, including weight reduction and increased physical activity. Cases of severe hypertension can be treated with medications. However, adolescent girls with severe hypertension should probably not be treated with drugs called angiotensin-converting enzyme inhibitors (or ACE inhibitors) because the medications can cause birth defects should a girl become pregnant.[10]

Stress can play a big role in the development of hypertension in teens. Girls who have chronic social problems, such as long-standing rivalries, struggles with parents to gain more freedom or to meet expectations in school performance can have chronically high blood pressure levels. The same effect is typically not seen in boys.

"Children with higher blood pressures tend to be the same people whose blood pressure will likely be in the abnormal or hypertensive range when they become adults."

—Dr. Michael A. Weber, American Society of
Hypertension

High cholesterol is another heart disease risk factor that should be treated promptly. According to the American Academy of Pediatrics, children over age two whose parents or grandparents had cardiovascular disease before age fifty-five or who have a history of cholesterol above 240 mg/dl are at risk for the disorder and should be screened regularly.[11] However, children without any risk factors need not be screened for high cholesterol.

Inaccuracies are common in routine cholesterol testing. For example, total cholesterol changes with age and can even differ by gender and race. To be more accurate, cholesterol levels should be tested several times and factors such as race should be considered. Children with confirmed high cholesterol can reduce their levels by adopting low-fat diets.[12] Parents need not worry that low-fat diets in children over age two will stunt growth in any way.

Cholesterol Levels for Children Ages Two to Eighteen from High-Risk Families:

	Acceptable	Borderline	High
Total Cholesterol	170 mg/dl or less	171 to 199	200 or more
LDL Cholesterol	110 or less	111 to 129	130 or more

Source: U.S. Department of Health and Human Services.

Reducing the Risk of Cancer

Cancer is such a horrible disease, and yet is so prevalent in our society that even very young children today often know it is a word to be feared—even if they don't understand just what it means. You can alleviate your daughter's fear of cancer by explaining what the disease is—simplistically, it is a disease in which cells in some part of the body grow uncontrollably—and the many ways in which she can reduce her risk for the disease.

The first fact that you will want to mention is that women themselves are responsible for astoundingly high rates of lung cancer and that those rates will be maintained or even climb if girls today continue to smoke in large numbers. Lung cancer is the most common cause of death from cancer among women, and it is due *almost entirely* to smoking.[13] Smoking also increases the risk of breast cancer by 25 percent.[14] The more cigarettes, the higher the risk.[15] However, women who quit can see their risk rates of all cancers drop back to that of nonsmokers.

Another form of cancer that may already be of major concern to your daughter is breast cancer. The dramatic women's health campaign in the 1980s and '90s to increase research on the diagnosis and treatment of breast cancer has brought the disease to the attention of even very young girls. If your family has a history of breast cancer, your daughter undoubtedly understands how devastating this disease can be.

But there are strategies to reduce the rate of breast cancer, which now affects about one in every eight women over the course of a lifetime.[16] It appears that a low-fat diet is important if it is started in childhood. While studies have found that women who adopt low-fat diets in middle age do not lower their risk of breast cancer, others have found that the diet adopted early in life does influence the processes that lead to cancer.[17] Most women get 30 percent to 35 percent of their calories from fat. A low-fat diet is considered one in which calories from fat do not exceed 20 percent. It is also abundantly clear that regular exercise over a lifetime significantly reduces the risk of breast cancer, as does maintaining a stable weight.[18]

Teenage girls are old enough to understand the high prevalence of breast cancer and learn what they can do about it. Before leaving for college, your daughter should know how to perform a breast self-exam.[19] Your daughter may be secretly worried about getting breast cancer if female relatives have been diagnosed with the disease. Increasingly, women who are at high risk for breast cancer are seeking counseling to help them understand their risk and deal positively with the fears associated with the threat of the disease. It's common for women with a high risk of the disease to exaggerate the risk in their own minds. Some women are so afraid, they cannot perform breast self-exams out of terror over what they might find. Louise, the mother of Missy, thirteen, explained breast cancer to her daughter when Missy's grandmother was diagnosed with the disease. "Missy is now aware of the risks. She clearly remembers Grandma's surgery and chemo. I think it's better that she understand what it is all about, even though the emotional side has taken its toll." Counseling can greatly help any woman, even your adolescent daughter, put her risk into realistic terms and learn how to live positively with the knowledge. If you (her mother) or a close female relative has had breast cancer, you need to spend time explaining the disease to your daughter in order to help her resolve her fears and give her the tools to better protect herself. Most breast cancer organizations have resources to help your family adjust to a breast cancer diagnosis (see Resources).

Ovarian cancer can have strong family links, although many women who develop the disease have no family history. There are a few things you can teach your daughter to lower her risk of this disease. One is the standard prevention advice to consume a good diet (low in fat and high in fruits and vegetables) and exercise regularly. Your daughter should also be told not to use talcum powder in the genital area because of some evidence that talcum powder can increase the risk of ovarian cancer. If your daughter likes to use powder, purchase a cornstarch product.[20]

NOTE: Health experts suggest that girls learn the acronym REMEM-BER as a guide to good breast health. REMEMBER stands for Risk Evaluation, Mammography Exam, Monthly Breast Exam, and Regular checkup. The risk evaluation part of the guidelines is a way for women to determine their risk of breast cancer by answering a series of questions that can help calculate their risk. These include the woman's age, history of breast cancer in her family, having had a breast biopsy showing abnormal cells, starting a period before age twelve, having a first child after age thirty or never.

Source: The Susan G. Koman Breast Cancer Foundation, May 4, 1999, REMEMBER Campaign.

Cervical cancer is another highly preventable disease. About 15,000 U.S. women are diagnosed each year, making it the second most common cancer in women.[21] The main cause of this disease is a sexually transmitted disease called human papillomavirus, or HPV. Up to 80 percent of women get HPV at some time during their lives, but only some strains of the virus cause cancer. HPV affects 13 percent to 46 percent of young women.[22] Cervical cell abnormalities are so high among girls today that health experts now recommend that all sexually active girls, no matter what age, undergo a yearly Pap smear.[23] Abnormal cells detected by Pap smears can be removed before they become malignant, but it's vital that HPV is detected early and treated. There is evidence that the virus causes the most damage in young girls compared to women.

Cervical cancer, if caught early, is highly treatable. But the disease can be fatal if it goes undetected for a long period of time and spreads to other organs. Sexually active teen girls should understand that they are at risk for HPV and cervical cancer and need to talk to their doctor about a Pap smear because the doctor may not mention it. One survey found that only 22 percent of women said their doctors talked about cervical cancer.[24]

> "Awareness and early detection are powerful tools in preventing cervical cancer. No woman should die of this preventable disease."
> —Dr. Sharyn Lenhart, past president, American Medical Women's Association

Skin cancer is also highly linked to behavior—the choice to be exposed to the sun without protection. White or fair-skinned people are most at risk and have twenty times greater risk for the disease. Following sun protection guidelines and performing skin self-exams periodically can greatly lower the death and trauma from this disease.[25] (See chapter 3 on skin care, for more information.)

Other Disorders to Be Aware Of

For many years, a heavy or abnormal menstrual cycle in girls was considered nothing to worry about. Now, however, enough research has been performed in women's health to know that menstrual cycle irregularities, even early in life, can indicate a possible problem. If your daughter has a heavy, painful, or irregular cycle, don't expect the worst. It may be that nothing is wrong and there is simply no cause or explanation. It's still a good idea to have these symptoms checked out by a gynecologist or endocrinologist, however. Heavy menstrual cycles can be an early sign of endometriosis, a condition in which excessive tissue grows around the female organs. Endometriosis is much more common in adult women. But since it can cause severe pain and infertility, it's important to have it diagnosed and treated as soon as possible.

Adolescent girls with irregular menstruation are also more likely to have a condition called polycystic ovaries. This is a disorder that causes the ovaries to produce excessive amounts of androgens. The ovaries can become enlarged and produce small cysts. Other symptoms of this condition may include acne, excessive body hair, and obesity. People with polycystic ovaries are also at higher risk of severe, early-onset heart disease and uterine cancer. Any of these symptoms linked to polycystic ovaries should lead you to seek a consultation with a specialist.[26]

Urinary tract infections are very common in girls and women. About 3 percent of girls have them by age eleven.[27] Infections often occur because bacteria from the skin around the rectum or vagina invades the urethra and bladder. Untreated infections can cause serious kidney problems.

The symptoms of a urinary tract infection are frequent urination, strong urge to urinate, burning or discomfort while urinating, sensation of incomplete voiding, bladder pain, fever, cloudy urine, or urine with a strong odor. Any of these symptoms should alert you to contact your pediatrician. Some girls are more prone to urinary tract infections than others. But all girls can learn simple steps to prevent infections.

Repeated urinary tract infections in childhood increases by about four times the risk of a serious kidney infection called pyelonephritis of pregnancy. This condition in pregnancy can cause complications that increase the risk of low birth weight and premature delivery. The message for parents is that if your daughter has a history of urinary tract infections in childhood, she should be told that this is important health history to remember and pass on to her gynecologist or obstetrician later in life when she is considering pregnancy or becomes pregnant.[28]

Urinary incontinence is a subject even adult women who have the problem don't like to discuss. Nevertheless, if you want to spare your daughter some possible misery later in life, it might be good to point out that this condition affects 10 percent to 20 percent of adult women (up to 40 percent of women over age sixty-five) and there are a few good tips that can be practiced over a girl's lifetime to prevent problems.[29] The best advice for girls is to learn that pelvic exercises, called kegel exercises, are the best way to prevent urinary incontinence. These contractions of the pelvic floor muscles will strengthen the muscles to prevent incontinence later in life, such as after having a baby. To explain the kegel exercise simply tell your daughter to try to shut off the flow of urine and then let it start again. This contracting of the muscles that control urine is the kegel exercise.

Tips to Prevent Urinary Infections

- Drink eight glasses or more of fluids every day.
- Don't hold your urine for a long time when your bladder is full.
- After urination, wipe with tissue from front to back—never from back to front.
- When urinating, sit on the toilet with your legs spread several inches so the flow of urine is not obstructed.
- Buy cotton underpants for your daughter and allow her to wear loose cotton pajama pants at night without wearing any underwear.
- Avoid bubble baths or bath soaps with chemical irritants.
- Avoid wearing tight clothing.

Source: Procter & Gamble Pharmaceuticals, June 1996; Dr. A. Barry Belman; American Urological Association.

Questions to Ask Your Doctor

- My daughter is overweight. Does this mean we should have her screened for high cholesterol and high blood pressure?
- My daughter had a cholesterol test that showed an elevated level. How reliable is this one test?
- What therapies are used for children who have mild hypertension?
- My adolescent daughter is very large-breasted. Does this mean she should start having mammograms sooner than recommended?
- My adolescent daughter smoked for two years but quit. Is she still at an increased risk for lung cancer later in life?
- I used talcum powder on my daughter as a baby and she used it until recently when we learned it wasn't a good choice. How worried should we be about the risk of ovarian cancer?

Resources

- The National Alliance of Breast Cancer Organizations offers information about all aspects of the disease. Call 212-889-0606 or visit www.nabco.org.
- The National Cervical Cancer Public Education Campaign has information on prevention, treatment, and diagnosis. Call 202-530-4884 or visit www.cervicalcancercampaign.org.
- For a brochure on the breast cancer awareness guidelines called REMEMBER, call the Susan G. Koman Foundation's help line at 800-IM-AWARE or visit the Koman Foundation web site at www.breastcancerinfo.com.
- Cancer Care, Inc. has a helpful guide for girls whose mothers are being treated for advanced breast cancer. It's called *A Shared Purpose: A Guide for Daughters Whose Mothers Have Advanced Breast Cancer,* and can be ordered by calling 800-813-HOPE or at the web site at www.cancercare.org.
- *Mom Has Breast Cancer* is a video for children that discusses how breast cancer makes children feel and act. It can be ordered through KIDSCOPE, 3400 Peachtree Road, Suite 703, Atlanta, GA 30326 or by visiting www.kidscope.org.
- Fact sheets for parents of children with urinary problems can be obtained by writing to: NKUDIC, ATTN: UIC, 3 Information Way, Bethesda, MD, 20892-3580. Or call 301-654-4415 or visit the web site at www.niddk.nih.gov.
- Information on heart disease and guidelines for screening tests can be located at www.nhlbi.nih.gov.
- A government report explaining high cholesterol in children and the current guidelines for treatment can be obtained from the National Heart, Lung and Blood Institute. Ask for NIH Publication No. 91-2732 (September 1991). Call 301-496-4236.
- A parent's guide entitled *Cholesterol in Children: Healthy Eating is a Family Affair* can be obtained from the federal government to

help you understand how you can lower cholesterol intake. Ask for NIH publication No. 92-3099 (November 1992). Call 301-496-4236.

- To better understand what is considered high blood pressure in children, you can obtain the most recent government guidelines on the topic, entitled *Update on the Task Force Report (1987) on High Blood Pressure in Children and Adolescents: A Working Group Report from the National High Blood Pressure Education Program*. Ask for NIH publication No. 96-3790 (September 1996). Call 301-496-4236.

- Two good guides for children and teens that explain the importance of a good diet to lower cholesterol intake are available from the federal government. *Your Health, Your Choice*, is for eleven- to fourteen-year-olds. Ask for NIH publication No. 98-3101 (April 1998). *Healthy Habits: Don't Eat Your Heart Out*, is for fifteen- to eighteen-year-olds. Ask for NIH publication No. 93-3102 (September 1993). Call 301-496-4236.

- For more information on urinary tract infections in girls, consult the American Urological Association's guidelines panel summary report on the management of primary vesicoureteral reflux in children. Visit www.auanet.org.

CHAPTER 10

Genetics: Clues in the Game of Health

W HEN DEBORAH looks at her daughters, Heather, sixteen, and Kelly, seven, she sees strong, fit, healthy girls with bright futures. Only one thing casts a shadow on Deborah's dreams for her daughters' futures, and that is her large family's history of breast cancer.

"Breast cancer is a huge problem on both sides of the family. I've had four aunts and my grandmother diagnosed with breast cancer. They have each had one breast removed. I don't worry about myself. But my girls are my life!" She tries to counteract her fears by educating her girls on all aspects of the disease. "I've discussed this a lot with my sixteen-year-old, stressing how important early detection is. She knows that if she ever feels the slightest lump in her breast, she is to tell me immediately. My seven-year-old knows what happened to her aunts and grandmother and constantly asks questions. I don't hold anything back when answering her. I believe that early detection is the thing that can save our lives if it happens to one of us."

Deborah's situation is a familiar one to many families. Over the past two decades, scientific research has made us much more aware that many diseases and disorders run in families. This knowledge is double-edged. While it can be frightening to know that we may be more susceptible to some illnesses, the knowledge can also be empowering because it gives us the opportunity to do something about the threat, such as learning about early symptoms or what we can do to prevent the disease.

The revolution in genetics will have a much greater impact on your daughter than on yourself, as scientific advances accumulate. At the start of the new century, we have enough knowledge to be convinced that the study of genetics will dramatically transform prevention and treatment of disease in the coming decades. Genes are the basic units of material that may be passed through generations of families. Each gene in the human body has a function, such as to create a particular eye color, fuel reactions between cells, or promote growth. Most human genes play a positive role in our health. But each person has genes that are flawed. These faulty genes can contribute or be the direct cause of disease. Estimates are that 30 to 50 percent of all childhood and 10 percent of all adult hospital admissions are related to genetic disorders or diseases. You are probably aware of genetic diseases that children are born with, such as cystic fibrosis or sickle cell anemia. But genetic-related disorders are not always apparent early in life. The onset of an inherited disease can occur later in childhood or, most commonly, in adulthood. These include adult-onset diabetes, breast cancer, and certain forms of heart disease.

Being informed about your family's patterns of illness will

be extremely important and helpful to you as the guardians of your daughter's health. For example, suppose you knew that your family had a history of speech and language disorders. Until recently, this fact would have been considered a curiosity. But, in 1999, researchers located a gene that is thought to be responsible for speech problems. Now, families with this history can be alert to take quick action should a child show signs of having speech or language problems.

Mental illnesses also tend to run in families, a fact that has become sharply apparent over the last few decades. The illness known as bipolar disorder has an especially strong familial link. Since bipolar illness usually first appears in the late teen years, knowing that your daughter may be at risk should help you prepare for the possibility. You should know what bipolar disorder is and what the early symptoms look like. As with many illnesses, the more quickly an individual is diagnosed and begins treatment, the better the chance that the illness can be quickly brought into control with minimal residual damage to the person and her life. Terri, whose husband, Pat, has bipolar disorder, has told her daughters, Shelby, ten, and Marla, seven, that the disease often occurs in families. "My husband turned fifty last year, and in March he was diagnosed with manic depression, or bipolar disorder. His behavior affected his job performance, relationship with friends, and especially our family. We discussed ways to tell what kind of mood Dad was in and what we can do to minimize the impact. I have discussed, and will continue to discuss, inherited traits—good and not so good," says Terri.

Patrice, mother of Ellie, nine, also says she will use her family's long history with mental illness as a tool to educate and protect her daughter. "I've struggled with depression from the time I was eleven. My mother and my mother's father were both institutionalized for mental illness at one point during adulthood. If my daughter shows signs of depression, I will take her to a doctor immediately and point out our family history: mother, grand-mother, great-grandfather—all with varying degrees of mental illness!"

Alcoholism is another extremely common disease with strong family patterns. If you recognize a prevalence of alco-holism in your family, it will be important to discuss this with your daughter so that she understands that the decision to drink might have deeper consequences in her life, compared to people who do not have a strong family history of alcoholism. Even minor con-ditions, like allergies or eczema (a condition causing dry, scaly skin) can have hereditary influences. Knowing about these condi-tions will allow you to respond quickly at the first sign of the problem in your daughter. You should also share your knowledge of your family's history of skin problems with your daughter's doctor, who might be aided in making a correct diagnosis.

Finally, many diseases with genetic origins are influenced by lifestyle factors, such as diet, exercise, and stress control. You can dramatically help your daughter alter her risk of some diseases by adhering to particular prevention strategies. LuAnn says that she pays close attention to her family's diet in order to lower the risk that she or her daughter, Trudi, six, will develop heart disease and diabetes. "These illnesses are very prevalent in my family," says LuAnn. "Trudi has already started learning about the risk factors that can be controlled."

Genetic information today has its limits, however. And, over the coming years, families will be faced with important, and sometimes very difficult, decisions about how much they want to know about their genetic legacy. An important national project, called the Human Genome Project, is nearing completion. This will give scientists a map of every one of the 100,000 or so genes in the human body. But even though new genes are being discov-ered almost daily, we still have few tools that can help us actually prevent or change the course of illness.

"Unfortunately, genetics is at an awkward stage, one in which the ability to predict diseases, in most instances, far precedes our ability to treat them."

—Raye Lynn Alford, *Genetics and Your Health*

What this means for parents is that you need to stay informed about scientific advances in genetics and educate yourself about genetic conditions that affect your family. You don't need to have a degree in science to do this. You only need to follow the news on gene discoveries and treatments that may pertain to your family's health history as well as asking your doctor to keep you informed. Part of your task to prepare for the revolution in genetics medicine is to do your best to comprise a family health history. And some genetic tests are available now that you may want to learn more about.

Keeping Your Daughter's Health History

Having a family health history will be increasingly important for your daughter as she grows up. If you don't have good records, construct a thorough history. It's most likely that you will be the first member of your family to establish this important tradition. If your daughter is old enough, ask her if she wants to help you gather information. This may help her better understand her own risks while giving her the feeling that she is doing something important to prevent disease in her life. Kashawna and her daughter, Kayla, fourteen, recently created a family health history as part of Kayla's science class homework. The project led mother and daughter into discussions about family matters that they had never discussed before. "My grandfather had diabetes. My father has bipolar disease. On my husband's side there is heart trouble," says Kashawna. "We've discussed what to watch out for in all of these areas. We've talked about the social stigma attached to mental illness, and she understands that it's a chemical imbalance that the person cannot control and is not to be blamed for."

To create your own family health history, start by interviewing relatives. Construct a family tree—geneticists call this a genogram or a pedigree—and write down such facts as how old relatives were when they died, what they died from (or what their symptoms were if there is no known cause of death) and what other illnesses they suffered from. If possible, find out the age of onset for the disease. Diseases that occur early in life tend to have stronger genetic roots. You can even try to track down death certificates or obtain old medical records. Try to find out something about the relative's lifestyle as well. Was the person overweight? Did the relative exercise, smoke, or drink? These lifestyle behaviors often make a big difference in the emergence of a genetic illness. For example, a family may have a predisposition to developing cancer. But someone in that family who smokes may be more likely to actually develop the disease.

Record information from parents, brothers, sisters, aunts, uncles, and cousins. For your daughter's pedigree it is especially important to have accurate information on the female relatives, particularly on the mother's side of the family.

All of this information will give you, and any doctors or genetic counselor you consult, a picture of the pattern of illness in your family. If certain risks appear, a doctor can advise you on whether your daughter should undergo screening tests to watch for early signs of the disease or on how to lower your daughter's risk through diet and exercise, which can have such a powerful impact on curbing a great many diseases. "My father died at age forty-eight of a heart attack. Since I am now forty-six, my daughter is aware of my father's death and she knows I try to watch the fat in my diet," says Carla, whose daughter is eleven. By being a good role model, Carla says she hopes her daughter will realize that she, too, can take steps to prevent disease.

Genetic Testing

There are now several tests available that can tell individuals if they carry a specific gene that is highly likely to lead to a particular disease. And, as the Human Genome Project is completed, the number of these tests is expected to grow dramatically. You need to understand the implications of genetic testing—especially in the context of what it could mean to your daughter. Genetic testing can give families vitally important information. Learning whether or not they carry a particular gene is empowering and can help families take actions to help lower their risk or detect the disease in its earliest stages. But there are also many good reasons to consider *not* having genetic testing.

One problem is that most tests predict only probabilities, not certainties. Another downside to testing is that knowledge of particular genetic traits can lead to job discrimination, insurance discrimination, or even discrimination against racial or ethnic groups (although laws exist to prevent this, including the federal Health Insurance Portability Act, which protects people in large group insurance plans from having a rate change because of a genetic test result).[1]

There may also be a high psychological price involved in genetic testing—and this is where you have to consider that any actions you take as parents may profoundly affect your daughter. Knowing that you carry a gene for a particular illness causes deep anxiety, even depression, in some adults. There is almost no understanding of how this kind of information could affect a developing girl. For example, what if a fifteen-year-old girl learns that her mother and aunts carry the genes for breast and ovarian cancer? She could begin to worry not only about her longevity but about how the possibility of disease could affect future relationships—even her decision to marry or have children. As parents, your job is to put your daughter's interests first—even before your own. Thus, if you are considering a genetic test for yourself, you need to consider what this knowledge may mean to your child. Charles, whose daughter is sixteen, says they both worry about their family's devastating pattern of early Alzhiemer's disease. What upsets them, says Charles, is that there is presently so little that can be done to change the course of the disease. "My daughter is aware of my family's history of Alzhiemer's disease, and it does frighten her," says Charles.

Health experts working on genetics understand the serious ethical and psychological issues that this new field of medicine will create. Much effort is being devoted to understanding how genetic information can be used positively while minimizing the negative consequences. To help parents, the American Society of Human Genetics and the American College of Medical Genetics issued a report on genetic testing in children and adolescents.[2] The report noted that genetic testing can have many negative implications for children. Thus, it advised that "timely medical benefit" should be the primary justification for having a child undergo a genetic test. For example, a family with a history of a heart disease that causes sudden death may benefit from knowing this and taking precautions. Or families with high cholesterol would benefit by starting their daughter on a special diet to reduce the consequences of the disorder.

However, if the benefits of having genetic knowledge will not be apparent until adulthood, then the report advises deferring the testing until the child is grown and can make her own decision. For example, the gene test that determines Huntington disease, a terrible condition that occurs around middle age and causes a severe decline in mental functions, would not be acceptable for use in a child since the symptoms and disease do not occur until adulthood and there is no intervention that could alter the course of the disease.

Children have a limited ability to understand disease and may even blame themselves for having genes that will lead to disease. They may lose self-esteem, become anxious about their future, and suffer a loss of privacy. A girl is likely to feel guilty should testing show a sibling has a genetic disorder but she does not. Parents need to seek counseling and give serious consideration to any form of genetic testing by any member of the family.

Specific Gene Tests to Consider

Perhaps the most important genetic discovery that may impact your daughter is the BRCA1 and BRCA2 genes, which play a role in the development of breast and ovarian cancer. There is still not a full understanding of what these genes do. But scientists believe that these two genes alone cause about 10 percent of the 180,000 cases of breast cancer diagnosed each year in the United States.[3] To put it another way, women in general have about a 10 percent chance of developing breast cancer before age eighty-five. But women with the BRCA1 or BRCA2 genes can have a 50 to 85 percent lifetime risk of breast cancer.

Ovarian cancer is also dramatically increased by the presence of these genes. A woman's normal lifetime risk of ovarian cancer is 1.4 percent. But the BRCA genes push the risk to a 15 to 45 percent chance over a lifetime.[4] The BRCA genes are most common among Jewish women, especially those of Ashkenazi descent.

What should you do if your family has a history of this

gene? As discussed above, your decision not only involves the mother, but the daughter as well. The daughter of a mother with a BRCA mutation has a 50 percent chance of inheriting that mutation. A granddaughter of someone with the mutation has a 25 percent of inheriting it.[5] Girls who know they have inherited this gene should be extremely vigilant in performing breast self-exams beginning at age eighteen, having breast exams by a doctor, and undergoing mammography beginning at about age twenty-five. There is also a medication for adult women called tamoxifen that can be taken to possibly reduce the risk.

For ovarian cancer, protective measures include being knowledgeable about the early symptoms of the disease (which are vague and difficult to detect); having regular examinations of the ovaries, including a pelvic ultrasound test; having blood screening tests for markers that may indicate the presence of ovarian cancer, and by taking oral contraceptives, which can cut a woman's chances of developing the cancer by at least 50 percent (more if the pill is taken for six or more years).

In cases where a family's history of breast or ovarian cancer is extreme, a woman may make the difficult decision to have the breasts and/or ovaries removed to prevent the growth of a tumor.

Colon cancer is another strongly genetic disease. About 5 to 10 percent of colon cancers are caused by a genetic mutation called HNPCC. Among people with this gene, the risk of developing colon cancer goes up dramatically. If the gene is present in your family, your daughter needs to know that she should undergo a colonoscopy, an examination to look for tumors, beginning around age twenty.[6]

As many as 50 percent of all heart disease cases also involve inherited gene mutations. Some prominent ones include the gene for hypercholesterolemia, which raises a woman's risk of heart disease to 50 percent over her lifetime. People with this gene can use diet, exercise, and medications to greatly lower their risk.

For now, the treatment of most genetic disorders involves dietary changes, surgery, or medications. In the future, gene therapy—the insertion of new genes into the body to take over for the flawed genes—may play a larger role in the treatment, and even prevention, of many diseases.

What a Genetic Counselor Does

If you are struggling to decide whether your family should undergo genetic testing, you don't have to sort through the complex issues alone. In fact, you shouldn't. There is a lot of uncertainty and sophisticated science behind the understanding of genetics, and experts in this field will be able to see a lot of things that won't be apparent to laypeople. Genetic counselors are trained to help families sort through information, better understand their risks, and make intelligent decisions on what will best benefit them.

The genetic counselor can give you a picture of the patterns of disease in your family and may also be able to give you an estimation of the "odds" that your daughter might develop a disorder. But the counselor should also explain any exceptions or special considerations that could alter this estimate. Moreover, the most important part of your discussion should include recommendations about what you can do for your daughter to alter her risk.

When it comes to your daughter's health, it is probably only necessary to seek genetic counseling if you or your spouse know or suspect you carry a gene for a serious disease or you know you have a family history of a serious disease. There are about 1,700 genetic counselors nationwide who belong to the National Society of Genetic Counselors. To find a counselor, call the society (see Resources), ask your doctor, or call a local university-affiliated hospital.

Questions to Ask Your Doctor

- I was diagnosed with breast cancer at age forty-one and there are two other second-degree relatives who have had the disease. Should I have my fifteen-year-old daughter tested for the BRCA genes?
- The heart condition called Long QT Syndrome appears to run in my large family. I would like to have my family tested, but my sixteen-year-old daughter resists the idea. How can I convince her? Should I demand that she be tested?
- My family has a long history of being overweight. Is this something that could have hereditary influences, and is there anything we can do about it?
- My ten-year-old daughter is extremely moody and cries a lot. There is a strong pattern of depression in my family. Should I be concerned that she could develop clinical depression and is there anything I can do right now to lower her risk?
- Can you recommend a good genetic counselor, and will my insurance cover the cost?

Resources

- To find a genetic counselor near you call a local university or contact the National Society of Genetic Counselors in Wallingford, PA. Call 610-872-7608 or visit its web site at www.nsgc.org.
- *Genetics and Your Health* by Raye Lynn Alford, Ph.D. (Medford Press, 1999) is a good guide to understanding genetic research and how it affects you.
- *Past Imperfect: How Tracing Your Family Medical History Can Save Your Life*, by Carol Daus (Santa Monica Press, 1999) explains genetic science and provides detailed instruction on how to obtain your family's health history.
- The National Foundation for Jewish Genetic Diseases provides

information to families of Eastern and Central European Jewish descent. The center is located at 250 Park Avenue, New York, NY 10017. Call 212-371-1030.

- The Alliance of Genetics Support Groups is a national coalition of professionals and consumers that voices the concerns of people living with or at risk for genetic conditions. The alliance is located at 35 Wisconsin Circle, Suite 440, Chevy Chase, MD 20015-7015. Call 800-336-GENE. Visit its web site at www.geneticalliance.org/.

- *Will I Get Breast Cancer? Questions and Answers for Teenage Girls,* by Carole G. Vogel (Julian Messner, 1995), is a wonderful book for teen girls who may be concerned about the disease.

- For information on the policies and progress of the National Human Genome Project, visit www.nhgri.nih.gov.

- For consumer information about the implications of the Human Genome Project and what it might mean to you, visit the Human Genome Project Information web site at www.ornl.gov/hgmis/resource/assist.html.

- The National Organization for Rare Disorders is a federation of more than 140 not-for-profit health organizations serving people with rare disorders and disabilities. The organization has information on rare diseases and where to find local support groups. Call 203-746-6518 or visit www.rarediseases.org/.

- Cancer and Genetics is an information resource to help people understand the genetic basis of cancer and interpret new genetic discoveries in the field of cancer. Visit www.cancergenetics.org/.

- *Genetic Testing for Breast Cancer: It's Your Choice* is an on-line brochure answering consumer questions about genetic testing for the disease. Visit www.cancernet.nci.nih.gov/genetics/breast.htm.

- *Genetics and Schizophrenia* is an on-line booklet for consumers. Visit www.nami.org/disorder/990305.html.

- Hadassah, the Women's Zionist Organization of America, offers instruction to show high school girls how to perform breast self-exams. Call 212-355-7900.

- You can send for a booklet entitled *Understanding Gene Testing*, published by the National Institutes of Health. Call 800-4-CANCER or fax your order to 301-330-7968.

CHAPTER 11

Reproductive Health: Biology, Sexuality, and Relationships

I'M AFRAID to talk to my parents about sex, because when I go on dates they're going to assume that I'm going to have sex," says Juanita, fifteen. "That's why I won't talk about it. And I'm worried that they're not going to know what to say or they will have some reaction like, 'Oh, my god, she wants to learn all those things about sex.' It's hard to look my mom in the eye and talk about things like that. She hasn't brought it up. So I just talk to my friends."

Juanita's parents may well be among those who feel over-whelmed by the responsibility to teach their children about sex. But sex is among the many topics that will require countless hours of conversation between you and your daughter. This isn't easy for many parents. Few of us were raised by parents who talked openly and repeatedly about healthy sexuality. Maureen is another parent who admits that she can't bring herself to discuss sex with daughter Lily, age thirteen. "It's too hard to bring the topic up. And it's too embarrassing. I wish I could talk to her about it."

Before talking to your daughter, you may first want to explore your own attitudes about sex. Carlene, whose daughter is nine, remembers her own uncomfortable relationship with her mother about matters of sex. "When I was pregnant with my third child, my mother was upset to hear my older sons talking about the baby in Mom's uterus, how the placenta works, and that the baby is born through Mom's vagina. She is very conservative and never discussed things like this with us when we were growing up. I think it's very important for children to realize what things are normal and not be afraid or embarrassed."

Ask yourself whether there are particular feelings or attitudes that you don't want to convey to your child. Will you feel too uncomfortable to do an adequate job? Like Juanita, many teenagers say the biggest barrier to effective parent–child communication about sex is the parents' lack of comfort with the subject. If you feel ill-prepared, there are programs and guides that can help tremendously. (See Resources.)

> "There are some bad things out there that girls get mixed up with. Not drugs or alcohol. People. Some people can get into really serious things and be tempted by boys."
> —"Girlfriend" on the World Wide Web

The risks our daughters face today are so widespread and perilous that it's essential to provide them with ample guidance beginning early in life. You are the primary sexuality educators of your children. Your goal should be to help your daughter become a sexually healthy adult. Each family will define that in its own way. But, for many parents, a central objective is to teach your daughter to feel proud and protective of her body, know how to set her own terms in a romantic relationship, and know the facts about reproductive health and staying free of disease and unintended pregnancy. Says Marissa, the mother of Daria: "We feel the main things she needs to know are that sex is great in a loving and committed relationship; how to protect herself against disease; her absolute right to say no; what it's like being pressured to have sex when she's not ready." To accomplish this kind of goal, however, you need to be astute about what kinds of pressures kids face today. Then look for opportunities to convey information, values, and expectations to your daughter. Be approachable so that she feels comfortable coming to you with questions. Callie, fourteen, looks proud when she describes how her parents have handled discussions about sex. "My mom is a nurse, and she knows a lot of things. I can talk to her about everything I want to. I don't even need to ask. They started to explain when I was little."

"I feel like if we start talking about it now, hopefully it will be natural to talk about it when she's older and facing those decisions," says Gerri, whose daughter, Allison, is eight. Gerri has the right idea. Talking about sex is easier if you start when your daughter is young. It's natural for younger children to be curious about their bodies. One of the best things you can do at this stage is remain relaxed and not get flustered when your daughter has a question about sex or her body. Jeanette, whose daughter is twelve, has found that starting young has helped both mother and daughter establish a connection on the topic. "We began when she was eight and have slowly progressed since then. She is very knowledgeable about many things. I help her by discussing things from a more clinical perspective. That made it easier on both of us to start that way. She continues to come to me with questions as things crop up." Give age-appropriate information. Think about what your child may really want at this particular moment. Is she asking for information? Making sure she is normal? Testing your knowledge? Exploring her values? Satisfying curiosity? The Sexuality Information and Education Council suggests parents keep this checklist in mind when their child has a question:[1]

1. Make sure you understand the question.
2. Think about what kind of message you want to give her.
3. Decide what response you want to give that will best represent your message.
4. Don't give more information than the child is really asking for at this time.

These guidelines can help you establish a good framework for future discussions with your daughter:

- By age five, she should be familiar with the correct terms for sexual body parts and know, in general, how babies are made.
- By ages six to eight, children should use the correct biological terms for body parts.
- By ages nine to eleven, children should know sexual feelings are normal and natural. They should have more detail about how babies are born, including how the reproductive cycle works. They should know that boys and girls undergo physical and emotional changes during puberty.
- By ages twelve to thirteen, children should understand that sexual relationships bring pleasure as well as a responsibility. They should know that abstinence is an excellent alternative for young people to remain healthy, safe, and strong. They should understand that there are serious consequences to sexual activity, including the loss of freedom from early childbearing. They should know how pregnancy can be prevented with different kinds of contraceptives.

They should know what sexually transmitted diseases are and how
they are prevented, transmitted, and treated.

Source: The Kaiser Family Foundation and Children Now, "Talking with Kids
about Tough Issues, 1999."

As your daughter gets older, she needs you to discuss this
topic with her as much as before—even if you've done a good
job providing information during the early years. If you don't feel
your daughter is asking enough, take the initiative and bring up
the topic. The ages of ten to fourteen are the key years to begin
discussing more complicated issues of sexuality (beyond what
preschoolers and young children ask while playing in the bath-
tub). Talking about sex means more than just doling out facts.
Your daughter needs to hear your thoughts about healthy relationships and values, too. Listen carefully to your daughter's concerns and questions. Try not to become threatened if her beliefs
are different than yours. Kids can act rebellious and defiant but
may actually be very frightened.[2] Loving support from parents
can make a big difference. While your daughter may now be getting more information about sex from the media and her friends,
parents are still the source of information kids most value.[3] "We
have stressed that this is a family subject and not to be shared with
friends," says Patrice, whose daughter, Diane, is eight. "Their parents will talk to them when they are ready. We have encouraged
her to ask us any question that she may have. We will be direct
and honest and will not be embarrassed."

Many surveys in recent years, however, show that parents are
not talking to their teenagers enough about sexuality and that
kids are turning more and more to TV for information.[4] Part of
this is natural. Girls are often spellbound by portrayals of romance
and sex on TV. Their fascination with sexual content on television has to do with the drama that surrounds the information,

says Jane Brown, a University of North Carolina researcher who has studied this topic.[5] "TV provides kids with the opportunity to see sexual scripts. They develop mental models about sex. While parents can talk about sex, television shows it to them. They see intimate things that they wouldn't see any other way." Jennifer, sixteen, says that when girls watch romantic situations on television they compare themselves to characters who are older than they are. "You see preteens reading *Seventeen* magazine because they want to be older. Teenagers watch *Friends* because they model themselves after people who are older."

For girls, says Brown, ages eleven to thirteen is the period when they are sensitive to these sexual scripts on TV. "They have characters they can identify with. They are looking for themselves. They are looking to answer questions they have themselves." Parents should monitor carefully the kinds of programs their children want to watch on TV. In some cases, it might be helpful to watch the program with your daughter and discuss what is going on.

"My daughter is a devout Christian and believes that she has to save herself for her husband. I am not crazy enough to think she won't change her mind and have discussed this with her also, explaining that she will know when the time is right. I don't want

FACT: Parents cannot rely on schools or physicians to provide their children with adequate information on sex. Schools are often guided by a program that reflects the politics or values of a particular interest group. Typically, the curriculum is based on abstinence only. Find out what your school is teaching. But remember that it will only be a tiny fraction of what your child needs to know and it's not coming from you—the person your child is most likely to listen to and believe in.

her to think she's forbidden to have sex, but on the other hand, I don't want her to become pregnant or get an STD. This is a very tough subject. But I think my daughter and I have a good enough relationship to talk things through. I also know she has a mind of her own and she's gonna do as she pleases. So I have tried to make sure she understands the risks involved. All I can do is pray that she has the presence of mind to remember what she has been taught in the heat of the moment!"

—Jill, mother of sixteen-year-old Kristen

Ben, whose daughter is nine, has come to grips with the main message he wants to give Melissa about sex. "The most important thing I think I can teach her is abstinence and that sex is best in a loving and committed relationship. She will also be taught about safe sex, in the event that she does decide to become sexually active."

One of parents' biggest fears is that talking to their kids about sex means you are giving them the information to go ahead and do it. Study after study has shown that this is not the case. Instead, parents who talk openly about sex and values are more likely to have teens who postpone sexual intercourse. Moreover, kids who are taught about both abstinence and contraceptive options are more likely to postpone having sex.[6] But when they do start having sex, they are more likely to use protection. It makes a lot of sense to view the matter this way: When you *don't* talk to your kids about all aspects of sex, the message you're giving them isn't that it's bad to have sex, it's that it's bad to plan for sex. Galina recently gave birth after becoming pregnant at sixteen. Her parents had never discussed sex with her. "I needed someone to tell me that it is normal to be curious about sex, but that you don't have to act on it. Just to be able to talk about sex and know that talking isn't a bad thing. If you are a teen and thinking about sex, you're considered bad. You're wrong. But kids need to know it's normal to think about sex."

Try to create an atmosphere in your home in which your daughter feels comfortable asking you anything about sex. Surveys show that even older teens have huge knowledge gaps about sex, including such facts as what is safe sex, what are emergency contraceptive pills, and how condoms are used.

> "The major message about sex education has to be clear, and it is: Don't have sex until you're ready. But if you do, use protection."
>
> —Ellen Wartella, communications researcher,
> University of Texas, Austin

Facts About Kids and Sex

Just over half of all high school girls say they have had sexual intercourse. Not surprisingly, a good many of them pay a price for becoming sexually active before they are ready. Consider these statistics:

- One million teenagers become pregnant each year; half of them give birth.[7]
- One in five girls use no method of contraception, which conveys a 90 percent chance of pregnancy over the course of a year.[8]
- Sexually transmitted diseases, including HIV, are spreading faster among young people ages ten to nineteen than among any other group.[9]
- In a single act of unprotected sex with an infected partner, there is a 30 percent risk of contracting genital herpes and a 50 percent chance of contracting gonorrhea.[10]
- Females are much more likely to contract gonorrhea, HIV, and herpes from a single act of unprotected intercourse than are males.[11]

- Females with STDs are less likely to have symptoms than males and thus may go undiagnosed and untreated while serious health problems develop.[12]
- Teens are more likely than adults to contract STDs because they tend to have more sexual partners.[13]
- Teenage girls are more susceptible to cervical infections from STDs than adult women because of their immature cervical anatomy.[14]
- When females get STDs, they suffer more effects than males. For example, girls with STDs increase their risk of becoming infertile and their susceptibility to certain reproductive cancers.[15]
- An estimated 15 percent of infertile American women have damaged fallopian tubes caused by pelvic inflammatory disease resulting from an STD.[16]

There are positive trends underway across the country, however, that should give you encouragement to continue talking to your daughter about sex and emphasizing your family's values. For example, the number of teens having sexual intercourse has not increased in the 1990s, and teen pregnancy rates have actually dropped.[17] Increasingly, the idea of remaining a virgin is acceptable to teens and is even admired.[18] Almost half of kids ages thirteen to eighteen now say they have made a conscious decision to delay intercourse. One in two teens say they have been in a situation where they could have had sex with someone they liked but decided not to. Surveys also show that teens are aware and do worry about pregnancy and HIV. Still, physical intimacy increases as teens age. By age seventeen, sexual intercourse is part of many teen dating relationships.

Making Good Decisions

Linda was sixteen when she became pregnant. A bright student and obedient daughter, she became pregnant the first time she had sex. Linda gave up her baby for adoption and, five years later, still cries softly over her youthful mistake. "I knew the facts. It wasn't a matter of being uneducated about sex. It was more because of the pressure from my boyfriend. You know, he'd say, 'If you love me, you'll do this.' I thought nothing bad would happen to me."

Linda's story illustrates the need for parents to discuss more than just the physical aspects of sex. Part of teaching your daughter about sexuality involves teaching her communication and decision-making skills that will help her in romantic relationships. Adolescent girls often have difficulty negotiating sexual situations. "We have spoken about the emotional involvement that should accompany sex," says Rhonda, the mother of Teresa, fourteen. "That means we have talked a lot about love and what it means to each person."

Teen girls are rarely encouraged to think about sexual situations in terms of their own desires. And, adolescents who are uncomfortable with their sexuality may have more trouble communicating their own wishes. In one survey, 61 percent of girls said that pressure from boys is often a reason girls have sex.[19] This is typically the kind of situation in which a girl is alone with an older boy in his home when his parents aren't there. Maria found that her relationship with an older man made it difficult for her to stand up for herself. "I was going out with a guy who was twenty-one, and I was fifteen. There was always trouble because he always wanted to have sex, and I didn't." Maria managed to get out of the relationship. But girls who are depressed, have low self-esteem, or feel a loss of control over their lives often find it much harder to stand up for themselves.

And they often regret their actions. Most teen girls who have had sex said they wish they had waited until they were older. Often this pressured, premature sexual activity leaves girls feeling abused because their expectations are so different from boys'. Dr.

Drew Pinsky, cohost of the radio and TV advice show *Loveline,* says that the most common destructive behavior he sees in today's youth culture is girls' willingness to forego their values, common sense, independence, power, and logical thinking in order to please a boy.[20] "For young women, disempowerment is a huge issue," Pinksy says. "The single most damaging thing I see is young women who are being asked to subjugate their values to a guy—even among women who are taught to be assertive."

Adults should probably ponder what the sexual revolution has really meant—and done—to our young girls. A single standard of sexuality shared by both men and women and emphasizing equal rights has replaced the old "double standard" that boys can be wild, while girls' virtue should be honored and protected. While this double standard of sexual behavior may seem old-fashioned and paternalistic, it afforded girls a measure of protection that, today, they clearly lack.

Some experts have referred to this cultural shift as "the demoralization of girlhood." In her book *A Return to Modesty,* the young writer Wendy Shalit argues that girls' lack of sexual modesty has led them into situations where they are no longer protected or respected.[21] She suggests that a single standard of sexuality for both males and females denies girls' true desires to engage in more meaningful sexual relationships than just the physical, one-night stands practiced by the current culture of young people. "Our culture gives women bad advice by encouraging promiscuity. Women are told that this is the road to equality, but that's a lie. Usually what happens is just the opposite. Women become more insecure. Modesty is a wonderful impulse that protects us," Shalit says. Perhaps Shalit's book represents a shift back to a more thoughtful, protective, and helpful way for girls to learn about their own sexuality.

In any case, your daughter will need guidance from you about how to handle sexual negotiations and continual reminders that her feelings and wishes matter. This is usually what kids mean when they say they are not getting enough information from their parents about sex. Eliza knows all too well the pressures that girls face. She was seventeen when she became pregnant with Jennifer, now ten. "We stress emotional preparedness and rules for dating, including the use of a chaperone," Eliza says. As part of that "emotional" preparedness, girls need to be taught that it's dangerous to offer token resistance (saying no to sex but not really being committed to stopping the sexual advance). If you feel you don't know how to provide this instruction, seek advice. Several communities have programs that teach negotiating skills in dating relationships. Also, Girls Inc., a national, nonprofit organization dedicated to helping girls plan successful lives, has a program called Will Power/Won't Power that helps girls practice these skills.

One of the most helpful things you can tell your daughter is that not all teens are having sex. Research has shown that teens who believe that at least some of their friends and peers are refraining from sex are far less likely to have sex themselves.[20]

> "The most corrosive thing we do is teach girls they have to be peacemakers. Those are the girls who find themselves caving in to pressure."
>
> —Caroline Miller, editor, *Seventeen* magazine

Certain situations clearly increase the odds that girls will engage in risky sexual behavior. Teens who drink alcohol, smoke, or use marijuana are more likely to be sexually active.[23] When drinking, teens are far less likely to use condoms. Girls whose families move frequently are at higher risk of premature sexual activity, too, possibly because the girl feels less support in the community, resents her parents for moving, and is acting out or is depressed or lonely.[24] Girls who have suffered sexual abuse are also far more likely to begin voluntary sexual activity at young ages.

If a Teen Is Sexually Active

Sexually active teens must have detailed information about all contraceptive options and have access to them. If you know or suspect your daughter is sexually active, make a concerted effort to obtain appropriate medical care. For example, federal health authorities now recommend that all sexually active teen girls should be tested *twice a year* for chlamydia, a type of sexually transmitted disease that can cause pelvic inflammatory disease and infertility.[24] Most sexually active girls are not getting anything close to adequate health care. A survey found that only one in four sexually active fifteen- to seventeen-year-olds reported every having been tested for HIV or any STD.[26]

Perhaps most importantly, sexually active teens should know about emergency contraceptives. Emergency contraceptives are ordinary birth control pills that can be taken up to seventy-two hours after unprotected intercourse to prevent pregnancy. Any doctor can prescribe emergency contraceptives by writing a prescription for a few birth control pills. There are also two brands of emergency contraceptives called Preven and Plan B. Girls or their parents can find a physician who is willing to write a prescription by calling the toll free emergency contraceptives hot line (888-NOT2LATE, or visiting the web site at www.NOT2LATE.com).

Questions to Ask Your Doctor

- Can my daughter confide in you about her sexual history and will you oversee her care or refer her to another doctor?
- I think my daughter is sexually active but am not sure. Can you talk to her about protection and test her for sexually transmitted diseases?
- Can you write a prescription for emergency contraceptives so that we can have it on hand at home?

- At what age should my daughter be seen by a gynecologist?
- Are there programs in my town that help girls learn how to negotiate sexual situations?
- Are there programs in my town to help parents learn how to talk to their kids about sex?
- I'm having trouble talking to my daughter about sex. What's a good way to begin the conversation?

Resources

- Sexuality Information and Education Council of the United States, 130 West Forty-second Street, Suite 350, New York, NY 10036-7802; www.siecus.org.
- *Talking About Sex: A Guide for Families* is a package containing a video, sixty-page Parent's Guide, and sixteen-page Children's Activity Workbook. Designed for parents with children ages ten to fourteen, it is available through Planned Parenthood, Inc., and can be ordered for about $30 plus shipping. Call 800-669-0156.
- A brochure entitled *Becoming An Askable Parent* can be obtained for $1 from the American Social Health Association at P.O. Box 13827, Research Triangle Park, NC 27709. Or call 919-361-8400.
- You can learn more about Preven emergency contraceptives by calling 888-PREVEN2 or visiting the web site at www.PREVEN.com.
- The National Campaign to Prevent Teen Pregnancy has a web site with information for both teens and parents. Access it at www.teenpregnancy.org/teen. You can order the campaign's free brochure, *Ten Tips for Parents to Help Their Children Avoid Teen Pregnancy*.
- Planned Parenthood provides information on sexual health, gynecological exams, pregnancy testing, and other issues on its site for teens at www.teenwire.com.

- The Kaiser Family Foundation has a web site for parents to help them talk to kids at www.talkingwithkids.org.
- Girls can call this toll-free number, 888-BE-SAFE-1, to request information on HIV, STDs, or to find a clinic for testing.
- A good book on girls and sexuality is *Venus in Blue Jeans*, by Nathalie Bartle (Dell, 1998).

CHAPTER 12

Preadolescence: Ages Ten through Twelve

Aᴍᴏᴛʜᴇʀ and her prepubertal daughter were visiting the pediatrician one day for a checkup when the doctor noticed acne on the girl's face.[1] Wondering whether the child was going to have an early puberty, the doctor asked the mother if her daughter had developed any other signs of puberty. The mother answered, "No," to which the daughter quickly responded: "But Mom, you told me I've developed an attitude!"

The years of ten to twelve are often delightful for girls and their parents. Children are beginning to learn responsibility, fairness, and to understand the need for rules. Meanwhile, they retain the openness and playfulness characteristic of their younger years.

But look closely and you'll see why the years of ten through twelve are recognized today as one of the most crucial developmental periods for humans, perhaps especially for girls. It used to be that the teenage years were the ones that sent parents reeling. But, notes Maura, whose daughter, Katie, is ten: "She hasn't had her period yet. But we're seeing great attitude changes, like bossiness and sloppiness. She wants to be treated like a queen." And, observes Michelle, whose daughter, Brandi, is eleven: "The past eighteen months her body has started to change. But in most ways, she's still a little girl. Her room is a marvelous cross between teddy bears and pop stars." Perhaps Kimberely, eleven, sums up this time of life best: "I think being a preteen is when you start thinking you're older, but you're still acting like a kid. It's a hard age to be. I want to do the stuff my sixteen-year-old sister does, and I'm too young."

With puberty occurring at much younger ages than ever before, preteen girls may have enormous trouble deciding whether they are "big" kids or still "little" kids. Physically, they may be rapidly growing up. But, emotionally, they are still very young. The outside world seems to treat these vulnerable girls as more mature than they really are. A lot of the risky behavior that used to be seen during the teen years is appearing in preteen youths. Preteens today are increasingly confronted by such serious issues as drugs, AIDS, and violence and trying to fit into peer groups. Faced with so many potentially heavy problems at such tender ages, many kids become anxious about their future. They are afraid they might use drugs, be physically or sexually abused or kidnapped, or might even die young. The collision of hormones, new pressures from the outside world, and the transition to middle school make this a time that requires great vigilance on your part as a parent. Girls at this age need to be protected, reassured, and encouraged.

The building blocks of early adolescence

This list describes the tasks that preteens should experience en route to a constructive adulthood.

- Find a valued place in a constructive group
- Learn how to form close, durable human relationships
- Earn a sense of worth as a person
- Achieve a reliable basis for making informed choices
- Express constructive curiosity and exploratory behavior
- Find ways of being useful to others
- Believe in a promising future with real opportunities
- Cultivate the inquiring and problem-solving habits of the mind necessary for lifelong learning and adaptability
- Learn to respect democratic values and responsible citizenship
- Build a healthy lifestyle

Source: 1995 "Report of the President," Carnegie Corporation of New York.

Physical Development

It used to be thought that nothing interesting was happening in the bodies of children between early childhood and puberty, Freud having labeled it the "latent" stage. But we know that hormonal changes may be taking place as young as six. Early secretions from the adrenal glands are among the first pubertal changes and these hormones, called androgens, may subtly influence behavior in kids ages seven, eight, or nine. If you think your ten-year-old daughter is showing signs of PMS, you may be somewhat correct in that hormones could be prompting behavior changes. This early sexual development is called *adrenarche* and is now thought to have a major influence on physical, emotional, and social development in middle childhood.

Body hair is often the first physical sign of adrenarche. "Even at not-quite-nine, her body is changing," says Leticia, the mother of Ally. "Breast development, getting curvier, oily hair, mood swings." If your daughter displays the first signs of puberty around six or seven, don't be alarmed. New guidelines by the American Academy of Pediatrics suggest such early development should now be considered normal and probably doesn't require an examination by an endocrinologist and any treatment to slow the onset of puberty (which was the common approach until recently for "precocious puberty"). What researchers are finding is that many more girls show the first signs of puberty at younger ages, but the process of puberty is actually spread out so that menstruation still doesn't begin for many until five or six years later.

But while early pubertal development may be normal, it doesn't make it any easier on a girl. The age at which your daughter reaches puberty can be of major significance. A girl may feel uneasy if she reaches puberty earlier or later than her peers. Girls who begin developing early tend to be at higher risk for problem behavior, including using drugs and alcohol at younger ages.[5] These risks do not arise from the early physical development but from the girl's tendency to hang out with older teens who may be experimenting with risky behaviors. Children who look older than they are may also be more likely to be left on their own after school.[6] Adults may treat these girls as being more mature than they actually are. That's what happened to Shelley, the daughter of Janet and Reggie: "Shelley has matured very fast. She resembles a nineteen-year-old right now (at age fourteen). The changes seemed to occur overnight somewhere between ten and thirteen. She had problems at school with socialization. Her teachers had problems relating her physical size to her emotional size. They assumed that she should know better, or be smarter, because she was taller by a good six inches than the tallest child in her class."

There are predictable stages, called the Tanner stages, to a girl's physical development that can stretch out over several years, beginning as early as age seven.

Stage I: No obvious sexual development.

Stage II: Rapid growth. Breast buds form. Some hair growth in the pubic and underarm areas.

Stage III: Breasts grow rapidly. Body hair continues to fill in. The clitoris grows. Menstruation can begin.

Stage IV: Breast and genital growth near completion. Menstruation has begun.

Stage V: Sexual development is complete and growth slows.

Menstruation

"I went to a school dance, and I started my period there. When I got home I was in the bathroom, and my mom was in there with me. Then my mom said, 'Oh my god, there's red.' I'm like, 'What?' What's wrong with me?' She yelled to my dad that I had started my period. I'm like, 'What?' I didn't know anything about periods. She had never talked to me. I was confused. Then my mom talked to me about it. She said once a month you're going to have this red thing."

—Heather, age twelve

Most girls begin menstruation between the ages of 11½ and 13½, or two years after the start of breast development. About half will get their periods by age 12½. Prepare your daughter for this event by explaining menstruation to her by age ten. Like Heather, Maricella is another girl who didn't learn about menstruation from her mother. Listen to how it made her feel: "My nineteen-year-old cousin asked me if I had started my period yet, and I said no. She went and told my mom to tell me about it. But my mom said no, that she would tell me when I started. It makes me feel like she doesn't really care about me or that I can't be close to her."

Whatever age your daughter begins menstruation, make an effort to frame the event in a positive light. The most central fact associated with women's health—hormone changes and menstruation—has, unfortunately, been viewed negatively in our culture, even by women. Parents today need to address whether focusing on menstrual disorders, such as premenstrual syndrome, unproved menstrual taboos, and pessimistic words such as "the curse" and "the rag" serve our daughters well.

There are certainly problems associated with periods, such as PMS or menstrual pain. But your daughter should receive positive messages from you about menstruation. She can be reminded that it is a sign of the very special function of women's bodies and that the hormonal shifts associated with menstruation are thought to confer very positive health benefits on women. Our daughters can learn that problems associated with menstruation can, and should, be successfully addressed.

Girls should understand the basic scientific facts of the menstrual cycle. The cycle begins on Day 1 with the start of bleeding and continues for about five days. From Day 5 until about Day 14, the body is releasing estrogen. Around Day 14, the ovaries release an egg; a process called ovulation. If the egg is fertilized with sperm, a pregnancy can occur. Otherwise, the egg simply travels out of the body with menstruation. From Day 14 until around Day 28, the lining of the uterus thickens with tissue and blood vessels to prepare for a pregnancy. Menstruation involves the shedding of that lining. Girls who have just started their periods need to know that it's not unusual to have an irregular menstrual cycle. It's often helpful for girls to keep a calendar of their menstrual periods in order to be aware of when the next one is due.

Girls need to learn good hygiene related to menstruation. Your daughter should be encouraged to try different pads or tampons until she finds a few products that work best for her. Many girls are most comfortable using different products for lighter and heavy menstrual flow. Girls need to know how to keep the genitals clean and to wash their hands before and after using menstrual products. Tampons should not be left in for more than a few hours.

Social and Emotional Changes

"I see my eleven-year-old getting moody and so I am afraid [puberty] is going to hit soon," says Mona. "She is a sweet girl but feels like the world is against her. I remember feeling that way. I am sometimes lost as to how to help her. She just wants to be liked so much." The very presence of hormones associated with puberty will introduce big changes in your daughter's behavior, as Mona has discovered. She will demonstrate a much wider range of moods and the ability to go from giddy to sorrowful in warp speed. While those mood swings are quite evident to parents—who may find themselves subjected to frequent demonstrations—girls, too, are very aware that something new and dramatic is happening. This realization can unsettle girls and cause them to become much more guarded and introspective. Girls may marvel at their new range of feelings but are unsure how to cope with those feelings.

Your daughter will begin showing the first signs of wanting independence, to be treated like a big kid, and to feel respected and responsible. Give your daughter increased responsibilities around the home. Encourage her to make choices and to fail. Praise her good choices and actions. Be aware that girls of this age seek independence but still can't control their impulses all that well. Girls having big problems may be more prone to run away during the early teen years more than any other time.

Girls who feel they can no longer connect with their parents may begin to withdraw. Crista, age twelve, is frustrated that she can't talk to her parents about the many questions she has. "Sometimes my parents don't understand what I'm going through. I don't have the confidence to tell them about boys and sex and other stuff. No one tells anyone anything in my family because there is this embarrassment."

Studies show that girls at this age begin to seek more time alone and desire more privacy.[7] They may also start to disagree more with their parents. If your daughter has been a child who readily complies with your requests, she may now start to ask more questions about why she should comply. It's important for parents to avoid being authoritarian ("Do what I say") and try to negotiate through differences.

You may notice a sudden desire to wear the latest clothing styles. Styles of dress and music are two of the main ways that preteens and teens express themselves and announce that gradual independence from their parents is beginning.[8] While you may not tolerate all of the choices they want to make, it's important to realize how important it is for girls to look and act like others. Try to understand your preteen's obsession with the physical and fashionable, but emphasize talents and character traits to downplay her interest in bodies and looks. Socially, this is an age in which peer pressure is extraordinarily powerful and the need to belong to a group especially acute. Patti noticed this about her daughter, Carrie, eleven. "She was very self-conscious and struggling to be herself yet remain part of her social group. She was not always happy about the new and difficult struggles she faced."

In fourth or fifth grade, the interactions between boys and

girls will also change as if "there is something new in the air," says Dr. Martha K. McClintock of the University of Chicago, a researcher of early puberty. For instance, boy-girl teasing may begin. While interactions between the sexes are not really sexual, she says, there is "a consciousness of liking and a recognition of vulnerability."

Relationship with Parents

Your daughter needs you now as much as ever. But at this age the need is different. Their need for love competes with their need to begin the journey toward independence. Studies show that up until age twelve, girls are very receptive to their parents' offers of support.[10] Sometimes, parents may forget how "little" a twelve-year-old really is. Notes Marcy, twelve: "Sometimes, my mother is like, 'Why don't you grow up? You act too much like a kid.' But I am a kid." Around age thirteen, kids become less confident in their parents' ability to help them.[11] For this reason, experts have referred to the age of twelve as parents' "last best chance" to reach out to their kids. You need to take every opportunity during these last years of complete childhood trust and openness to talk to your daughter about the issues that lie ahead.

> "My dad and I are really close. We think the same. We go fishing. When we're fishing, it's, like, special time together. We talk about sex and boys and drugs."
>
> —Leeza, twelve

After age thirteen, it often becomes harder for girls and their parents to communicate as openly. One study found that while just 23 percent of kids in fifth, six, and seventh grades said they were uncomfortable talking to their parents about sensitive issues, that figure jumped to 43 percent among eighth graders.[12] By thirteen, kids are more likely to say their parents do not love them as much, do not treat them with respect, and show less interest in talking to them. Some preteens said they want to talk to their parents, but can't because they are too busy. Even parents who were actively involved in their daughter's elementary school may find themselves uninterested in middle school life.

However, this is not a good time to draw back from your daughter's world. For girls, in particular, the transition from grade school to middle school or junior high, with its peer pressures and exposure to risky behaviors, makes this a very difficult time—one during which you must make a concerted effort to stay engaged with your daughter. It's sometimes helpful to guide your daughter into supportive environments that reinforce your family's values, such as church youth groups, girls' clubs, scouting organizations, or school groups. Surviving these years with a close relationship to your daughter is like money in the bank.

Questions to Ask Your Doctor

- My daughter has gained weight suddenly this past year. Does this mean her period will start soon?
- Is there any way to predict when my daughter may start her period?
- My daughter has frequent crying jags. Is this normal?
- What can be done to help my daughter with menstrual cramps?
- Should girls this age get treatment for what seems to be severe PMS?

Resources

- KidsPeace offers several pamphlets to parents on parenting, helping kids through crisis, and to preteens, including *What Every Preteen Wants You To Know . . . But May Not Tell You*. Its web site is at www.kidspeace.org/or call 800-8KID-123.

- A good book explaining puberty is *It's Perfectly Normal: Growing Up, Changing Bodies, Sex and Sexual Health*, by Robie Harris (Candlewick Press, 1994).
- Another good selection to help explain the physical changes of puberty is *What's Happening to My Body? Book for Girls,* by Lynda Madaras (Newmarket Press, 1988).
- *Keep Talking: A Mother-Daughter Guide to the Pre-Teen Years*, by Lynda Madison (Andrews and McMeel, 1997), is a terrific guide to staying close to your daughter through the crucial preteen years. It's geared to both mothers and daughters who can share the book and discuss its ideas and information.
- Playtex Products, Inc. has a twenty-minute educational video and information kit for girls focusing on menstruation. The cost is $7.95. You can order it by calling 877-4PLAYTEX or at www.playtextam-pons.com.
- For information on talking to your daughter about physical changes and sexual development, contact the Sexual Information Education Council of the United States (SIECUS), 130 West Forty-second Street, Suite 350, New York, NY 10036-7802 or call 212-819-9770.
- *The Girls' Guide to Life*, by Catherine Dee (Little, Brown, 1997), is a wonderful workbook to help girls navigate the social and emotional changes that accompany puberty.
- *Changes in You and Me*, by Paulette Bourgeois and Dr. Martin Wolfish (Andrews and McMeel, 1994), is another good book focusing on the physical changes associated with puberty.

CHAPTER 13

Adolescence:
The Growing-up Years

I KINDA FEEL in between childhood and adulthood," says Melissa, fifteen. "I know I'm an adolescent, but I like to think of myself as an adult. I enjoy having conversations with adults and talking to people about the news and weather. I baby-sit for a one-month-old baby and have even learned the responsibilities of that."

If you're like a lot of parents, you're probably dreading "the teen years." But you may find that the old idea that teenagers are loaded with emotional storms, angst, and serious misbehavior is a myth. While the preteen years and the transitional year of thirteen may indeed be rocky, most kids navigate adolescence without major problems.[1] Yes, your daughter will probably want less to do with you and will still have fits of moodiness and dejection. But girls are not bucking to cut off their ties to their parents so much as to redefine them. There is a big difference between wanting to become autonomous (which they desire) and wanting to separate (which they don't). Like Melissa's connection with the adults in her life, you may find yourself learning to talk and behave with your daughter in a much more mature way—one that honors the adult that she is rapidly becoming.

> "One myth says the goal of adolescence is to separate from your daughter. We see it another way. The goal is to build a strong relationship with your daughter, based on her evolving differently . . . adolescent girls want to be seen and heard for who they are and trusted with the truth."
>
> —from *Girls Seen and Heard,*
> The Ms. Foundation for Women

Thirteen: The Toughest Year

The early teen years are the most difficult for girls because it is then that they are making the transition from childhood to youth. Part of the challenges girls face during this time is simply hormonal—their bodies are pumping out hormones that can trigger emotional outbursts or crying jags. They may become so interested in boys that it seems as if all their other interests are forgotten. Whatever they're feeling, those feelings will be strong. Chris, the mother of fourteen-year-old Megan, puts it another way. "Ages ten to twelve were hard—moody—but nothing like thirteen!" Ruth, the mother of Ashley, saw age thirteen as a bizarre blip in her daughter's development. "She had always been extremely shy until she reached thirteen. She became very demanding at school, very disrespectful of the teachers at school, and aggravated me to death with her attitude. When she got out of eighth grade, she calmed right down again."

Dealing with the hormone-driven storms of this period will require you to have patience and to keep your own emotions in check. You need to remember that your daughter is more confused than you are about what is happening to her and her body. If you maintain a warm, supportive relationship with your daughter, she will lower her defenses and will be less afraid to confide in you. You need to also remember that this period doesn't last forever. In another year or so, you will be amazed at your daughter's maturation. Now that Miranda is sixteen, her mother Ann is feeling pretty good. Miranda is smart, talks openly with her mother about all kinds of things, and is only slightly moody at times. "She is well-informed and has appropriate values," Ann muses. "I think my biggest concern is social skills, having friends that don't exploit you and tell tales about you and have stupid values."

> "Scratch that adolescent attitude and you'll still find your daughter underneath, as much (if not more) in need as she ever was of being reassured in word and deed that she's one of a kind and dear to your heart."
>
> —*Girls Seen and Heard,* The Ms. Foundation
> for Women

What Teens Are Up To

Adolescent girls are experimenting with different roles. They are struggling with social pressures and learning how to handle various peer situations. They are trying to figure out where they fit in in the world. They are trying to establish an identity while constantly making self-observations and comparing those observations with their peers. For girls who are adopted, the search for an identity may suddenly cause problems with their earlier acceptance of adoption.[2]

Your teenager may spend a fair amount of time belittling or hating herself—something you need to tune into and counter with positive messages and by teaching your daughter to think positively about herself. A teen girl's thoughts, feelings, and plans can be expected to change from day to day. Indeed, ambivalence about everything in her life may be the hallmark of your daughter's behavior for a good stretch of adolescence.

Your daughter may also start spending, or wanting to spend, a lot of time away from home. One estimate suggested that a high school senior spends 60 percent less time at home than she did as a fifth grader.[3] You might be upset about this and think it suggests rejection of the family. It doesn't. It simply means that your daughter is growing up. Sometimes, teens will seem to be trying to push their parents away. "I see her at school and she is talking all the time and yet in the car she is so quiet. I wish I could read her mind," notes Lydia of her teenage daughter. Because the hours spent with your daughter will decline, you need to be ready to listen and take advantage of those dwindling opportunities to talk to her. Those discussions will probably be on your daughter's timetable—and at some horribly inconvenient time for you! While it may seem as if girls are more comfortable talking to their mothers, they still need the counseling and love of their fathers. Ron, the father of several teen girls, says that he tries to encourage his daughters to confide in him about the problems and issues in their lives while letting them know that he expects them to abide by the family's values and rules, such as arriving home in the evening by a certain hour. "Girls need respect and honesty as they grow. They need a dad who is a 'safe' man. A dad needs to be there to gently redirect any inappropriate behaviors."

Socializing will become extremely important to your daughter, and you may find yourself grappling with setting up new household rules for where she can go, with whom, and for how long. Teens can enjoy social situations safely as long as some planning goes into the events. It's up to you to make sure that any parties your daughter is attending are safe and supervised. Don't rely on schools or other parents to do this for you. Poorly planned parties in which parents have turned a blind eye to the event sometimes result in tragedy.

A Safe Teen Party Guide

If your teenager is attending a party, consider these guidelines to ensure safety:

- Know where she will be. That includes the name of the host, address, and phone number. Tell your daughter that she has to inform you if the party location changes.
- Contact the parents of the party-giver. Verify that the party is taking place at the location given. Make sure an adult will be present and offer assistance. Make sure drugs or alcohol won't be permitted.
- Know how your daughter will get to and from the party. Discuss transportation and make sure your teen knows she can call you for a ride. Make sure she has a phone number to call in an emergency and discuss situations in which your daughter might want to call you or use the emergency contact number (such as if the friend who is driving has consumed alcohol).
- Make an agreement on when your daughter is expected home. Be aware when she comes home or have her wake you up. Take a few minutes to talk to your daughter when she gets home to find out how the evening went. If the party involves overnight arrangements, make sure the plans are discussed in detail with the host.

If you and your daughter are hosting a party:

- Set the ground rules before the party. This means sharing responsibility for the party with your daughter and letting her know what you expect.
- Be home during the party. Take the time to meet your daughter's friends. Arrange for the party to take place where you can adequately supervise it. Never allow a party to take place when you're not there. Inform neighbors of the party.
- Limit the party attendance and times. Plan the party by issuing invitations. Don't let the group get too large. Set time limits to avoid open-ended parties. Discourage teens from leaving the party to go elsewhere and return.
- Don't serve alcohol to anyone under age twenty-one. Don't have any alcohol in your home that is easily available. Be alert to signs of alcohol use by other teens. Notify the parents of a teen who arrives at the party under the influence of drugs or alcohol.

Source: Napa Police Department and Napa Valley Unified School District.

Parenting a teenager involves the delicate balance of continuing to protect her while allowing her to assume more responsibility for herself. Your daughter will need your acknowledgment that she is growing up. Girls who are overly controlled by their parents and feel no power themselves may turn inward to something they can control, such as eating, leading to abnormal behavior and mental health disorders like anorexia.[4] Indeed, the struggle between a girl's desire for independence and her parents' desires to protect her will be most acute during the mid to late teen years. Female teens, very much like their male counterparts, will have a sense of immortality and a belief that nothing bad can happen—good reason for you to continue to stand firm where safety is a concern.

Teenage girls often fail to grasp the huge risks that substance abuse, early sexual activity, and other dangerous behaviors entail. You must realize that how your daughter copes with the risks of adolescence depends very much on her disposition, her environment, and your family. Girls who are living in dysfunctional families can be expected to have a much harder time surviving adolescence in good physical and psychological health.[5] Indeed, when major difficulties arise in adolescence, it is often due to a teenager's surroundings, particularly if her environment is a troubled one. Teenage girls who are dealing with poverty, their parents' troubled marriages, neighborhoods or schools where they are victimized, or the community's ambivalence toward youth may turn out to be the unruly teens that seem so unapproachable.[6]

> "Parents need to know that the process of kids withdrawing from family life is very typical. There will be fewer times when a son or daughter will just plop down in the living room; instead they will be withdrawing to the bedrooms or going off with friends."
>
> —Reed Larson, psychologist, University of Illinois

The "Ophelia" Phenomenon

In 1994, the brilliant psychologist Mary Pipher gave parents of girls a plateful to think about with her best-selling book *Reviving Ophelia*.[7] In it, Pipher describes how many girls go from confident and happy to lost and sad in the years between ten and fourteen. They turn sullen and self-critical. Their grades drop. They stop caring about things. They hate their bodies. Pipher blames this phenomenon largely on American culture: the "sexism, capitalism, and lookism," which evaluates a person based only on appearance.

Aimee, fourteen, notes how changing bodies captures great

attention. "Puberty is a big deal and scary," she says. "People make fun of others for the way they're developing. I think kids worry because they know they're growing up."

Girls sense that they are not safe in a culture that does not value their true selves. They grow silent and confused, often until late adolescence when new skills help them emerge with a strong sense of personal identity. While all girls in adolescence experience periods of doubt and despair, you can help your daughter stay true to herself by talking to her about her thoughts and feelings and helping her understand her life. Encourage your daughter to ponder her problems, write in diaries or journals, seek advice from others, and resolve to figure out the puzzles in her life. According to Pipher, one of the most important questions girls need to ask themselves repeatedly during adolescence is " 'Who are you?' The answer is beside the point," Pipher says. "It is the process a girl goes through attempting to answer that question that keeps her in touch with her feelings, experiences, goals, and dreams and puts into place the role of her family, environment, and culture."

> "Certain kinds of homes help girls hold on to their true selves. These homes offer girls both protection and challenges. These are the homes that offer girls affection and structure. Girls hear the message, 'I love you, but I have expectations.'"
>
> —Mary Pipher, author of *Reviving Ophelia*

The Question of Peers

Friends become very important during the adolescent years. You should make a big effort to get to know your daughter's friends and to speak up when you are concerned over the influence a friend may be having. Girls do influence one another in major ways. According to a study, peer "pressure" is just the tip of the iceberg.[8] This study found that:

1. Peers offer models of how to act and what to believe.
2. Peers create situations that allow for good or bad behavior (for instance, hosting parties when parents aren't home).
3. Peers set standards of behavior and attitudes—or norms—for each other.
4. Best friends and the leading crowd at school are less influential than most people assume. The friends who are the most influential regarding the timing of first intercourse and the risk of pregnancy are the five to ten friends in a girl's immediate circle and the fifty or so larger group of friends and associates.
5. In general, a teen girl's low-risk or "good" friends seem to help more than the high-risk or "bad" friends seem to harm. The presence of a number of low-risk friends in a girl's circle, for example, significantly decreases her chances of becoming sexually active or pregnant.
6. Peer influence can increase the risk of early sexual activity, particularly if a teen girl associates with older kids—male or female.
7. While a girl's relationship with her parents is important to such things as reducing her risk of early sexual activity, equally important is the relationship that a girl's close friends have with *their own* parents.

Let your daughter know that you are also interested in her friends and in their lives. Open your house to your daughter's friends so that you can get an idea of what they are like and how they interact. If you have a concern about a friend, don't order your daughter to stop seeing the person. But talk to her about the friend and let her know of your concerns. If your daughter is in a school club, sport, or any type of organization, volunteer to be a parent helper or chaperone. What your daughter doesn't tell you about her life may be apparent if you look closely enough at her environment. Above all, reassure your daughter that you trust her ability to choose her friends wisely.

Advice for Parents About Peer Pressure

- Look beyond your child's best friend to her wider network to understand the full range of peer influence.
- Encourage your teen daughter to spend time with low-risk friends. They make a big difference.
- Discourage your teen from hanging out with older kids.
- Learn more about how your daughter's friends get along with their parents.

Source: "Peer Potential: Making the Most of How Teens Influence Each Other" and "Power in Numbers: Peer Effects on Adolescent Girls' Sexual Debut and Pregnancy."

Teens and Sleep

One of the ironies of adolescence is that just when your daughter is looking more grown up, she regresses when it comes to sleep. Many parents, and even health professionals, are surprised to learn that teenagers need more sleep than their younger siblings. Puberty triggers big changes to a teenager's internal body clock. Teens often have difficulty falling asleep before 11 P.M. Many will even lie awake until 1 A.M. or so. But they need to sleep longer than younger children—about nine hours and fifteen minutes a night to be truly rested.

The problem is that few teens get this much sleep. Typically, a teenager will stay up very late and then will have to wake up very early to get to high school classes that begin, in some schools, as early as 7 A.M. As a result, many teenagers are horribly sleep deprived and pay a high price for their fatigue. About 23 percent of teenagers report being tired during the day.[10] Tired teenagers get sick much more frequently, have trouble studying, and are less in control of their emotions and moods. Some even fall asleep in school.

It may be tough to do much about this situation, especially if your school starts early and if your daughter has to rise early on weekends for a job or extracurricular activity. You can try to convince your district school board to move back the school starting time; an approach that has been tried occasionally around the country. If that fails, help your daughter take small steps that might gradually increase her sleep. These tips from the National Sleep Foundation include:

- Go to sleep fifteen minutes earlier each day and wake up fifteen minutes later until you are getting about nine hours of sleep. Avoid naps while in this process. This gradual shifting of sleep and wake times might shift the internal body clock and make it easier for teens to fall asleep earlier.
- Avoid caffeine or any stimulants in the evening.
- Avoid bright light in the evening.
- Relax before bed. Avoid heavy studying or computer games before bed.
- Don't go to sleep more than one hour later on the weekends than you do during the week.
- Do not go off schedule more than two nights in a row.
- Don't sleep in more than two or three hours past your normal wake-up time on weekends.

Questions to Ask Your Doctor

- My daughter sleeps until noon or one on weekends. Could this signify a health problem?
- When should my daughter begin seeing an adult doctor?
- My daughter spends a lot of time in her room by herself. Is this normal?
- What is an appropriate curfew hour for my daughter, given her age?

- My daughter is struggling with peers, school, and her feelings. Can you recommend a therapist she would be comfortable with?

Resources

- The T-Room is an interactive web site sponsored by Tampax that addresses menstruation and physical changes that girls undergo in puberty. Visit www.tampax.com.
- *Seen and Heard* is a book featuring essays by American adolescents, edited by Mary Motley Kalergis (Stewart, Tabori & Chang Publishers, 1998). To order call 800-BOOKS-NOW.
- A good book for girls on the *A* to *Zs* of adolescence is *Finding Our Way: The Teen Girls' Survival Guide,* by Allison Abner and Linda Villarosa (HarperPerennial, 1995). The book is especially sensitive to racial and ethnic differences among girls.
- *My Feelings, My Self*, by Lynda Madaras (Newmarket Press, 1993), is a workbook aimed at helping teens explore their thoughts and feelings. Lynda Madaras is also the author of *What's Happening to My Body? Book for Girls.*

CHAPTER 14

Mental Health:
A New Understanding

IT HAS BEEN thirty years, but Rosie still remembers how her life changed at the tender age of twelve. She became mentally ill. But no one noticed.

"That winter became one long term in hell. I wrote a lot of sad poetry and long rants in my journal, had a long unrequited love interest in the boy across the street, and basically had nothing I liked to do. My family teased me relentlessly about crying. I slept a whole lot. Food became a real interest," she recalls.

Rosie was on a decades' long downward spiral stemming from an untreated depression. She became bulimic and then began to act out by using drugs, drinking, and having sex. The drugs and drinking, she noticed, seemed to temporarily soothe her vicious moods. Rosie was smart and managed to perform well in high school. She graduated from college with honors. However, her demons did not abate.

"Fear and sadness tormented me. I wasn't treated for depression until I was thirty-one. At the time, I had a two-year-old, a newborn, and my husband had just had major back surgery. I simply cracked under the pressure. I remember rolling around on the floor, wailing. I went to see my doctor, who prescribed Effexor (an antidepressant). The medication changed my life. I cannot describe the different perspective I have on how I deal with stress, or how much more joyful my everyday life is now. I have lost a lot of my fear of living and have given up alcohol. The only feeling I have about the time I lost is regret that I didn't have the chance to get treatment much, much sooner."

When Rosie was growing up, it was uncommon for people to talk about mental illness. It was even less common for people to recognize mental illness in a child. Today, we know a lot more about mental illness. We know that it does not arise from personality shortcomings or moral weaknesses. Mental illness is, in fact, a brain-based disease that causes deep pain and suffering if it goes untreated. Slowly, the stigma attached to mental illness is fading away. More adults are talking openly about their own experiences with mental illness and are getting treatment. More children, too, are being properly diagnosed and treated for mental illness, although there are still a lot of people who believe, erroneously, that children do not become mentally ill. The truth is, many mental illnesses in adults probably had their beginnings in childhood or adolescence. As parents, you will be doing your child an enormous service if you understand, watch for, and respond to any signs of mental illness. All families should discuss mental illness and promote the idea that seeking help for these brain-based disorders is nothing to be ashamed of. As parents, we have the opportunity, for the first time in history, to raise a generation of children who are enlightened about mental illness and know what actions to take if it occurs in them or their future families.

> "If you're an adult with a psychiatric problem, there's a good chance that your problem started in some form when you were a kid."
>
> —Dr. Daniel Pine, New York Psychiatric
> Institute

Parents often blame themselves or wonder what they did wrong when their child is diagnosed with a mental illness. However, mental illness is rarely caused by just one thing. In all likelihood, a combination of factors leads to mental illness, including family dysfunction, a traumatic event, or genetic influences.[1] Hormones are also thought to contribute to some mental disorders in women. For example, by the end of adolescence, girls have two to three times' higher rates of depression than boys. And the rate of depression in girls doubles in the year after the start of menstruation.[2]

Stress

> "In my last year of junior high, my five-month-old sister died. And then my mom and dad got separated. Then they got back together again, and now my mom is pregnant. I started getting Ds and Fs on my report card. There was too much to deal with. I have so much responsibility at home. I am the 'mom' at home from 3 to 7 P.M. I try to talk to my friends about it. It gets a lot of the weight off my shoulders."
>
> —Janelle, age sixteen

Stress is not a mental illness. But stress can contribute or exacerbate mental illnesses. Because of this, you should monitor the amount of stress your daughter appears to be under and help her learn to cope with it in healthy ways.

Stress is a part of life, even the lives of children.[3] Like the stress that adults face, children under stress can react positively or negatively. And, like adults, negative reactions to stress are likely to have bad outcomes for children. As parents, your job is to help your daughter deal with stress in ways that leave her feeling more empowered, competent, and in control.

Perhaps the most important discovery in the past two decades about girls and mental health is that girls experience stress differently than boys. And the way girls absorb stress leaves them more prone to other mental illnesses; in particular, depression and anxiety. Rebecca saw this happen to her daughter, Melinda, fifteen, after the family suffered a series of blows. "At one point, we went through a very rough period as a family," Rebecca says. "Melinda's father was diagnosed with cancer, and we later separated. Melinda became very withdrawn and refused to talk about it."

A primary cause of stress among girls is relationships— between girls and their parents, girls and their friends, girls and their teachers. Because girls are socialized to be more sensitive and caring, problems in relationships take a much bigger toll on them.[4] It's for this very reason that Crystal and Mike say they will keep a sharp eye on their daughter, Amanda, even though she is only eight and is "a very sunny little girl." A few things worry the couple anyway, says Crystal. "Depression is very strong in my family. I suffer from it, as well as my oldest son. And Amanda tends to put a lot of importance on what other people think of her. This worries me that she may, in the future, tie her self-esteem to other people's opinions instead of believing in herself."

Because girls tend to feel responsibility for the relationships around them, they may react more harshly to divorce than do boys. Divorce is one of the most common, traumatic events that cause children enormous stress and that can pave the way to the development of depression.[5] If you are experiencing divorce, consider counseling to help your daughter. There are also some terrific books for girls on divorce (see Resources).

Death, injury, and sickness to loved ones can also precipitate high levels of stress, and even depression, in girls. American adults are often not good role models for healthy grieving. We also may not realize that children need mechanisms and rituals to mourn. We shouldn't try to shield or protect kids from grief and loss. Learning to deal with grief in a healthy way is a necessary part of growing up. But children don't always let us know when they are grieving. We have to be available to talk to them and listen to them. You can also help your daughter cope by allowing her to attend funerals and wakes and by allowing her to cry and ask questions. One way to start practicing healthy coping mechanisms in times of grief is to allow your daughter to plan a memorial service and burial when a pet dies.

Stress can also build as a result of daily life. Stress in girls, particularly adolescent girls, is often due to four powerful forces, according to research from Girls Inc.

- The battle of the body: As a girl reaches puberty, her changing body sabotages her. Just when she learns that thin, lean, and angular is supposedly the way to be, her body starts adding fat and curves.
- Wanting to conform when everyone looks different: Right at the time when a girl has a strong desire to conform, gain popularity, and peer acceptance, she looks around her and sees her classmates developing at hugely different levels and speeds.
- Searching for identity when the options conflict: As a girl approaches womanhood, she faces conflicting expectations for

what it means to be a woman today and the fact that she is grow-ing up to be a less valued member of society.

- Coping with new, unfamiliar, and unsafe environments: Changing schools, changing relationships with parents, and the personal risk of living in a violent and sexist society make her environment more stressful.

Another difference in girls is that they tend to internalize their emotions, while boys use more externalizing strategies. Girls, for example, may withdraw and worry silently, while boys will act out their stress. Chelsea, twelve, is typical in that, on the verge of adolescence, she has found herself changing in the way she handles stress by being more self-conscious about how she fits in and compares to other girls. "I use sports to keep from getting too stressed out, but sometimes people say I shouldn't be athletic. I play tackle football and sometimes the cheerleaders will make fun of me and the other girls who like to play hard."

Handling stress in a positive manner is crucial for good health. In children and teens, stress can contribute to depression, anxiety, eating disorders, smoking, drinking, and drug use.

How can you help your daughter avoid these dangerous and unhealthy coping mechanisms? First, address the areas that are likely to cause stress in your child (see Helping Your Daughter Handle Stress). Second, teach your daughter coping mechanisms to deal with stress.[6] Don't shield her from life's challenges, but acknowledge what she is facing and encourage her to cope in ways that build her confidence. Be warm and supportive of your daughter. Your reaction to your daughter's stress can have a big impact on how she faces challenges. Says Renee, eleven, "I don't get too stressed out because I get along really well with both my parents, especially my mom. She does so much and we can always talk to each other. I think she's great."[7]

Helping Your Daughter Handle Stress

- Help girls find their own skills and interests. One of the best ways for girls to become stress resistant is by having hobbies and skills and by placing a high value on them.
- Praise girls for what they do, not what they look like. If girls gain confidence from their skills rather than their appearance, they'll be less likely to be preoccupied with their own body images.
- Demystify puberty. Honest discussions about the changes girls experience will enable them to manage those changes more successfully. Start the dialogue early so girls and adults become comfortable discussing complicated issues.
- Equalize the chores. Be sure that girls aren't bearing disproportionate responsibility for child care and housework.
- Be a nonconformist. Celebrate your individuality. Talk freely about how you have set and met your own expectations rather than those of others.
- Dispel the myths. Smart women do get the guys. Beauty comes in many shapes and sizes.
- Label mixed messages so girls recognize that they don't have to do it all. Help them make the best choices for themselves.
- Encourage girls to build stress-resistant lifestyles by limiting caffeine intake, eating regular and nutritious meals, and building exercise into daily life.

Source: Girls Inc.

Depression

Tricia, twelve, seems very depressed, says her mother, Penny. "She is arguing with her friends a lot and feels as if no one likes her anymore and that the teachers have it in for her. She was a straight A student, but her grades have dropped. I don't know what to do with her."

Depression can occur in people of all ages, beginning in early childhood. Depression in children prior to puberty is uncommon—but it does occur. Families who are under stress due to divorce, moving, job or income changes, death in the family, and other major events are more likely to have depressed kids. Sometimes the typical events of adolescence can plunge vulnerable girls into real depression. "I had a boyfriend, but then we broke up," says Chloe, fourteen. "I was so depressed. I was like, oh my god, he left me. I stopped eating. I just lost my appetite." Fortunately, Chloe's feelings began to improve after two months. She regained her weight and suffered no long-term consequences from the depression.

Families with a history of depression should also be more cognizant that depression can arise in children at even young ages. A child with one depressed parent has double the chance of becoming depressed. Depression also tends to emerge at earlier ages when a parent has experienced depression.

Other risk factors for depression include dieting, which has been found to contribute to depression in girls.[8] Sexually active teen girls are also more likely to be depressed, possibly because they are conforming to what males expect of them and feel insecure and unprotected. Punitive parenting styles tend to aggravate the risk of depression in girls.[9]

In younger children, depression is often missed. Children ages six to eight with depression don't exhibit the same kinds of symptoms as depressed teens or adults. Children are typically happy. Indeed, if there is one key characteristic of childhood, it is

---

FACT: About one in every thirty-three children has depression. About one in eight adolescents has depression.

—National Mental Health Association.

joy. Thus, the lack of happiness, often expressed as apathy or boredom, may be a characteristic of depression in young children. They are likely to act aggressively or withdraw or complain a lot, especially about physical symptoms.

Children ages nine to twelve who are depressed are more likely to daydream, have morbid thoughts, and worry excessively.[10] In general, pre-adolescent children with depression are irritable, have problems with friends, and complain that others don't like them.

Depression in adolescents tends to resemble the symptoms seen in adults. It often shows up in school problems, relationship troubles, chronic feelings of guilt, changes in sleep or appetite, fatigue, and loss of interest in activities that were once enjoyable.

Perhaps the most difficult situation for parents is determining the difference between actual depression and normal teenage angst and moodiness. Look for three clues: how long the behavior has been going on, how intense the behavior seems, and how unusual your child is acting compared to her "normal" self.[11]

- Time: Any constellation of depressive symptoms that lasts beyond two weeks should start to concern you.
- Intensity: Ask yourself if your daughter's crying, rebellion, lethargy—whatever the symptoms—are occasional or constitute regular behavior.
- Comparison: Consider whether your child has gradually been shifting into this pattern or whether it has come on suddenly. A sudden onset is more typical of clinical depression.

If you're not sure if your daughter's behavior constitutes clinical depression, don't hesitate to consult with a medical expert. Even low-level, chronic unhappiness can increase your daughter's risk for a major depressive illness later in life.

The risks of depression are serious and often long-lasting. Girls who are depressed are more likely to have accidents, become pregnant, drink, smoke, and use drugs. About one in three depressed adolescents has thoughts of suicide. The combination of depression and substance abuse is an especially dangerous one that raises the risk of suicide.[12] Depressed children and teens have a higher rate of having other disorders, such as attention deficit disorder, conduct disorder, or eating disorders. The existence of more than one mental health disorder is called a "coexisting" condition.

Grief

Childhood is not very light-hearted and carefree for many kids. In fact, it is common for children today to go through a period of grief, either due to death or divorce. Adolescence, for example, is a period with a high death rate. Your daughter might experience the loss of a friend or classmate. More typically, she will lose a grandparent during childhood. Divorce, too, typically triggers a grieflike reaction in children. The grief of divorce is particularly profound if one parent deserts the family.

There may be little you can do about the causes of grief. But you can do a great deal to help your daughter learn how to experience grief in a healthy manner. This isn't easy for many parents because few of us were raised in homes where death and grief were confronted and discussed openly. Make a commitment to change old family patterns that deny or hide grief. Talk to your child about her grief and let her know that it is a normal reaction. Teach her how to say good-bye and resolve a loss in her life. Learning this in childhood will help her deal positively with inevitable losses and grief later in life. Take the time to learn about how children experience loss and what to do when they are having trouble recovering. Grief counselors can be located in

Depression and Risky Behaviors

High school age girls with depressive symptoms are twice as likely to smoke, drink, or use drugs.

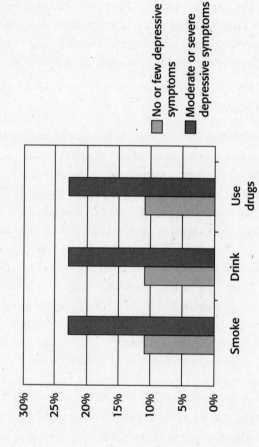

No or few depressive symptoms

Moderate or severe depressive symptoms

Source: Commonwealth Fund.

most cities and many good books for children of all ages are available on grief and mourning (see Resources).

Anxiety Disorders

When Keely was seven she had a tonsillectomy. The surgery went well, but what happened afterward alarmed her mother, Lynn. "After she had her tonsils out she started having anxiety attacks. She even had them at school. She was put on a medication, Paxil, to treat it. We were all very concerned. That is over now, thankfully. But it will be something that I will talk to her about a great deal as she gets older."

Most children become nervous or anxious before certain big events, like an important test at school, a piano recital, or a championship sports contest. But chronic, persistent anxiety that occurs for no apparent reason can signal the onset of an anxiety disorder. An estimated 5 percent to 10 percent of children have anxiety disorders.[13] Children with anxiety disorders will often try to hide their symptoms and have trouble articulating how they feel. The best clue to a problem may be seen in their actions, such as feeling too sick to go to school or refusal to go places or get involved in activities.

There are several kinds of anxiety disorders. They include: panic disorder, obsessive-compulsive disorder, post-traumatic stress disorder, phobias, and generalized anxiety disorder. Here is a brief explanation of each.

- Panic disorder: Feelings of terror that strike suddenly and repeatedly. These attacks cause heart palpitations, dizziness, stomach pain, shortness of breath, and a fear of dying. Women are twice as likely to experience panic disorder.
- Obsessive-compulsive disorder (OCD): Repeated, intrusive, and unwanted thoughts or rituals, such as repeatedly washing one's hands. OCD often begins in adolescence.

- Post-traumatic stress disorder: A chronic recurrence of symptoms that occur after a traumatic event, such as a rape, car accident, shooting, or earthquake. The person experiences nightmares, depression, and relives the feelings associated with the trauma.
- Phobia: An extreme, irrational fear of something that actually poses very little or no danger. People with a phobia go out of their way to avoid the object they fear. Social phobias—fear of interacting with people—typically begin in childhood.
- Generalized anxiety disorder: Chronic anxiety that accompanies everyday life and persists for a period of six months or more. People who are always anxious often have headaches, insomnia, fatigue, muscle tension, and nausea. Generalized anxiety disorder usually begins in childhood or adolescence.

You can see from this list that many disorders first emerge in childhood or adolescence. However, many people do not get help until they are adults. Panic attacks, in particular, often occur in girls around the onset of puberty. While girls may not develop a full-blown disorder until adulthood, early treatment of occasional panic attacks would help greatly to reduce the risk of a serious disorder later in life because girls can learn actions to take to stop the attack (such as breathing exercises to prevent hyperventilating).

Suicide

Life had not been easy for McKenzie. At thirteen, she was living with her father and stepmother, Bob and Joyce. At age ten, she was sexually abused by her mother's boyfriend. By age twelve, McKenzie was clinically depressed and began to talk about killing herself. "She initially told her godmother" about the suicide plans, says Joyce. "She had been spending the weekend there. Her godmother is a very good friend of mine and is also a social worker. Apparently, McKenzie told her that sometimes she just wanted to kill herself and that she would take pills or hang herself from the top bunk with a belt. With that degree of planning and forethought, I took it very seriously. We first went to our family doctor, who referred us to a walk-in psychiatric clinic at the university hospital. I took her there and found them to be utterly useless. The psychologist we saw minimized the whole experience. He asked her what she had said, why she said it, and whether she had 'learned her lesson.' He then went on to suggest that maybe I should see someone there, as I was emotional. I explained that I felt emotional was an appropriate response from a mother in this situation. We then took her to a see a psychologist through Catholic Social Services. He was a little more helpful, but mainly worked with her father and me. It seemed as though no one wanted to touch this kid with this issue. We worked through this on our own with her. Of course, we removed all medications and belts. We were always watchful."

Joyce and Bob recognized what many people—even therapists—don't: Children can become extremely depressed and try to kill themselves.

While suicide rates haven't changed much among adults over the past several decades, they have gone up dramatically in adolescents, and a depressed teen is as likely to commit suicide as a depressed adult.[14] Teens with depression or manic depression are at the highest risk of suicide. Suicide attempts can occur after a stressful event, such as an argument or humiliation. Drug use increases the risk for committing suicide. Depressed children who also have severe anxiety are at the highest risk of suicide.[15]

> "A few weeks ago I felt like ending my life because I thought no one liked me. But it was the exact opposite. The afternoon I was going to take a knife to my throat, my best friend came over. She gave me a blue ribbon that said, "Who you are makes a difference." She told

me I had made a good impact on her life and that I was her best
friend ever. I don't feel like dying any more."

—Brenda, fifteen

Adults often miss the warning signs of suicide. Girls considering suicide may say things such as, "I'd be better off dead,"
or, "Nothing matters any more." They may even talk about
their plans to commit suicide. They feel hopeless and alone.
They may give away favorite possessions, write good-bye notes
or poems to loved ones, or even say good-bye to friends. The
most vulnerable time for suicide occurs after a child has
endured a loss or humiliation, such as the breakup with a
boyfriend or being the victim of abuse or a prank at school. A
child may try to kill herself following a friend's suicide. Girls,
like boys, appear particularly vulnerable to suicide after an
encounter with the law.[16]

It's crucial that you teach your child that a friend's threat of
suicide should be taken seriously and reported to an adult, even if
it was told in secrecy. A poll found that 60 percent of teens have
known someone who has attempted suicide.[17]

What to Do When a Child Talks about Suicide

- Talk and listen to your daughter. Take what she says seriously
  and give her your full attention.
- Tell your child that she is loved. Point out all the people she has
  to turn to and who care about her, love her, and will help her.
- Don't try to tell your child that she has lots of reasons to live.
  Instead, acknowledge her pain and reassure her that she will
  feel better with help, support, and treatment.
- Get help immediately. Don't wait to see what happens. Contact
  an organization in the Resources section.

Getting Help

All mental health disorders can be treated. Some people and illnesses are more responsive to treatment than others. With children and teenagers, it's important to seek treatment as soon as possible after the illness has begun. Treatment often works better the earlier the illness is diagnosed. About two-thirds of mentally ill children do not get any help.

Andrea was eight when her older cousin, whom she was extremely close to, died of cancer. The incident plunged her into a clinical depression, says her mother, Katie. "When her cousin died, she had lots of loving support from her family, but since we were all going through our own kind of pain and mourning, it was difficult to know how to help her. I saw signs of depression: changes in behavior, she became quieter and less happy and bubbly. She was just different. Fortunately, she had a sensitive, caring teacher who also noticed the differences and suggested we see the school psychologist. After doing so, we agreed that my daughter would go for a visit with her during recess period. It was the best thing we ever did. They handled it so beautifully so as not to make her stand out or appear different in any way. The psychologist used art therapy techniques, which worked well since Andrea has artistic talent. She was able to express some of the feelings she had been unable to articulate." In a very short time, Andrea was herself again, says Katie. "She still wonders why her cousin died, but she deals with it by talking with me and writing her heart out."

Help is available. However, knowledge of childhood mental disorders lags behind that of adults' and is plagued with more questions than answers. Treatment of children is often difficult because they have trouble expressing what they are feeling and thinking and describing their experiences.[18] Moreover, knowledge about medications to treat children has advanced very slowly because of fears that the drugs might harm developing children.

What Can Parents Do?

- Be aware of the behaviors that concern you, note how long the behaviors have been going on, and how often and how severe they seem.
- See a mental health professional or the child's doctor for evaluation and diagnosis.
- Get accurate information from libraries, hot lines, and other sources.
- Ask questions about treatments and services.
- Talk to other families in your community.
- Find family network organizations.
- If you are not satisfied with the mental health care you are receiving, discuss your concerns with your health care provider, ask for information, and seek help from other sources.

Source: National Mental Health Association.

Treatment varies according to the disease, the severity of the disease, and other factors. In general, however, mental disorders are treated with some form of counseling or psychotherapy. There are also many good medications available, although many of them have not been tested specifically for children. Treatment for mental health problems can come from a variety of sources, such as social workers, family therapists, psychologists, and psychiatrists. It is also not uncommon for a child to have two professionals overseeing her care; for example, a family therapist to provide counseling and a medical doctor who prescribes medication. Look for a therapist who specializes in working with children, such as a licensed child psychologist or child psychiatrist.

It may not be easy to convince your child to go to treatment. Lindsay, sixteen, was asked to join her parents, Bill and Margie, at sessions with a counselor after the couple concluded that they were not dealing effectively with Lindsay's rebellious behavior. "She was acting obnoxious and saying things that alienated people from her," says Margie. "I have mild depression and yell at my children more than I should. Both their father and I (especially him) tend to be critical, although we say positive things, too. My daughter has been to a counselor with us, but she hates it and considers it a punishment. Later, I got her a kid's book on depression, and I think she found that helpful. The idea of the book is that these sad and bad moods are a physical condition and something that some people have to deal with."

Sometimes a family's treatment efforts are hampered because they find out that their health insurance policies have severe limits on mental health treatment. Because mental disorders are now considered to be brain-based biological illnesses, many Americans feel the reduced insurance coverage of mental health disorders is discriminatory and wrong. In many states, mental health activists are fighting for "parity," the equal coverage of mental illnesses alongside other physiological illnesses. If your child needs treatment, find out right away what your policy covers. At your first visit with a health care provider, discuss your policy and ask the therapist what he or she can do to help you make the most of your coverage. You can locate therapists who charge fees based on a family's income by calling your county mental health association. If you have a strong family history of mental health disorders, it may be prudent to consider arming yourself with a good policy—just in case.

Questions to Ask Your Doctor

- My daughter is fourteen and has had frequent crying jags over the last few months. She is very moody and stays in her room most of the time. How do I know if this is depression and needs treatment?

- I am concerned about my daughter's unrealistic fears of new social situations. How can I help her be more comfortable in new settings?
- I know my daughter needs therapy but my insurance will not cover mental health treatment. Is there a clinic that will accept us free of charge or on a sliding-scale fee structure?
- My daughter complains about her male therapist and says she would feel more comfortable talking to a woman. Should I change doctors?
- My family has a very strong history of bipolar disorder. What are the early warning signs of this illness, and is there anything I can do to help prevent it in my child?
- Our family would benefit enormously from therapy but my teenager refuses to go. How can I persuade her to go to therapy?

Resources

- Two useful books to help parents teach their kids lifelong stress-management skills are *Stress-Proofing Your Child,* by Sheldon Lewis and Sheila Kay Lewis (Bantam Books, 1996), and *KidStress,* by Georgia Witkin, Ph.D. (Viking, 1999).
- A good book on depression in childhood is *Help Me, I'm Sad,* by David G. Fassler, M.D., and Lynne S. Dumas (Penguin, 1987). Another guide for depressed teens is *When Nothing Matters Anymore,* by Bev Cobaine (Free Spirit Publishing, Inc., 1999).
- Parents with depressed adolescents should read *Understanding Your Teenager's Depression*, by Kathleen McCoy, Ph.D. (Perigee, 1994).
- Families who are considering therapy but have no clue what to expect can learn much about the process through the book *Behind the One-Way Mirror: Psychotherapy and Children*, by Katharine Davis Fishman (Bantam, 1995).

- A very helpful book for children about mental illness is *Know About Mental Illness,* by Margaret O. Hyde and Dr. Elizabeth H. Forsyth (Walker & Co., 1996).
- For information on mental illness, contact the National Mental Health Association at 800-969-NMHA. Another good resource is the National Alliance for the Mentally Ill, at 800-950-NAMI.
- A free brochure designed to guide parents in helping their mentally ill child can be obtained from the American Psychological Association at 877-603-4000.
- The New York University Child Study center has a comprehensive web site about the understanding and treatment of mental health disorders in children and adolescents. The site is meant to help kids, parents, educators, and mental health experts and covers topics from attention deficit disorder to anxiety, depression, social phobia, parenting, and more. Visit www.AboutOurKids.org.
- The American Academy of Pediatrics has a free brochure called *Surviving: Coping with Adolescent Depression and Suicide*. Visit www.aap.org.
- *A Girls' Guide to Divorce and Stepfamilies*, from American Girl Library (Pleasant Company, 1999) is a positive approach to helping girls deal realistically and constructively with the issues.
- Some helpful books on grief include: *Talking With Children About Loss*, by Maria Trozzi (Perigree, 1999); *When Someone Dies*, by Sharon Greenlee (Peachtree Publishers, 1992); and *Straight Talk About Death for Teenagers*, by Earl A. Grollman (Beacon Press, 1993).

CHAPTER 15

Violence and Personal Safety:
Smart, Not Vulnerable

Janice was fifteen and had barely begun to date when she met nineteen-year-old Colin. He was charming and good-looking—and trouble. Within a few weeks of their first date, Janice began to see flashes of Colin's terrible temper. When he became angry at her—for arriving late to a date or disagreeing with his opinions—he screamed at her, shoved and slapped her. During one argument, he broke her nose. "I was so in fear of him," says Janice, now eighteen. "I wanted to get out of the relationship, but I thought it was a matter of him trying to kill me." Janice became pregnant and wanted to have an abortion, which Colin objected to. Five months into the pregnancy, Colin was sentenced to prison for auto theft. Janice gave birth and turned her baby over for adoption. She and her mother moved to another city and, at last, Janice became free of the abusive man.

"I never wanted to get pregnant. I wanted to break up with him. But he was so threatening."

Your daughter will probably—and hopefully—never be exposed to a horrible act of violence. But don't wait until it happens to speak to her about it. Violence is an issue you must discuss with your daughter. This can be difficult, because many parents grew up in much safer environments, where dating violence was unheard of, where kids could freely roam their neighborhoods and towns or could walk to school without worry. It's hard to admit to ourselves that our children are not as safe. But with the widespread availability of guns and the prevalence of domestic and dating violence, the world today is a much different and dangerous place. According to the National Education Association, about 100,000 students carry guns to school. Homicide is the second-leading cause of death for women ages fifteen to twenty-four.

Talk to your daughter about how violence starts. Ask her how kids get along with one another at school and if they treat one another well. Listen to what your daughter says about her world so that you can help her form a response to threatening or potentially dangerous situations.

> "Parents should talk to their children about troublesome classmates, but also about their fears and the complex social situations that can lead to violence."
>
> —Dr. Ernest Fruge, psychologist and expert on
> violence, Baylor College of Medicine

Teaching your daughter to protect herself starts in very small ways, such as learning that her body belongs to her and she is its sole guardian. It means learning to respect her instincts when they tell her that a situation could be dangerous. It means learning to be assertive and bold when it comes to saying "no" to someone.

Your daughter should be aware of her vulnerability without feeling like a victim waiting to happen.[1] She doesn't need to be rescued, and in fact, you won't be there to rescue her in all dangerous situations. So teach her to respond on her own behalf. "I try not to frighten them about our society," says Cris, whose daughters are thirteen and sixteen. "I think bad things happen to people no matter what precautions we take, yet it is not healthy to overemphasize this. But they have been taught never to go with anyone, to yell really loud, and resist anything scary. The youngest is trained in tae kwon do and has an attitude to match!"

Scaring your daughter won't work. What she needs is a realistic view of the world and the skills and confidence to protect herself. This can be done by keeping excessive worries to yourself and emphasizing practical, everyday stuff, such as basic safety rules. This includes walking with buddies, not using a public restroom alone, knowing how to dial 911, locking doors, assessing an environment before entering it, and not opening the door for a stranger.

Be honest about violence, or your daughter may envision things as being worse than they really are. Let her talk about her fears and what has upset her. Overall, violent crime among all age groups has declined in the United States in recent years. Children need to know this kind of positive fact while being reminded of ways to avoid being a victim of violence. Brad and Donna have talked to their daughter, Lauren, fourteen, about safety issues since she was four. "When she was younger and wanted to walk to school alone and I wouldn't let her, she thought I didn't trust her. I told her that I trusted her; it was the strangers I didn't trust. We've talked about all kinds of abuse. We've also told her that if she is in an unsafe or uncomfortable situation to just call home and we will come and get her. Children need to have a safety net, and I think parents are to provide it."

Violence in the Media

"I do get concerned about my safety because I have seen the news and have seen what some people can do," says Olivia, fifteen. Hearing about violence and crime on television and other news programs can cause children to become fearful, sad, and depressed. Be aware of the content of news programs and turn off the television or radio, or discuss the content with your daughter to help put the news in proper perspective. Limit your daughter's exposure to violence in the media. Sit with her and explain that while most TV characters who are shot heal and return to normal, in real life people usually die or are permanently maimed by guns. Studies show children can become desensitized to violence and even believe that it is a normal response. Don't let your daughter talk you into letting her watch violent programs because all her friends are supposedly doing it. Tell her you are imposing rules on what she watches because you don't like the message that violence sends.

It takes work and planning to monitor your daughter's exposure to violence. Follow these tips from the Kaiser Family Foundation.

- Actively supervise your child's exposure to all forms of media violence.
- Limit TV viewing to those programs you feel are appropriate.
- Be selective about which movies your child sees and which video and computer games she plays.
- Establish rules about the Internet by going on-line together to choose sites that are appropriate and fun for your child.

- Consider using monitoring tools for TV and the Internet, like the V-chip.
- Take advantage of the ratings system that provides parents with information about the content of a TV program or movie.

You have two tools to help you monitor your daughter's exposure to violence on television: the V-chip and the TV ratings system. The ratings system, while far from perfect, will let you know whom the show is meant for and whether it contains violence, sexual situations, crude or profane language, suggestive language, or fantasy violence. The system doesn't do any good unless you monitor ratings and enforce the rules in your home. The V-chip is built into newer televisions and monitors the ratings so that you can automatically block out shows with certain content.

If you're like many parents, you probably consider the Internet a great tool to advance your daughter's education. Having computer and Internet skills are vital, as we shall see in the chapter on education. But the Internet has a huge downside. Unsupervised use could expose your daughter to dangerous and harmful material, including pornography, material demeaning to women, propaganda, and the glamorization of violence. One poll found that 44 percent of teens had seen X-rated web sites or sites that contained sexual content, and 25 percent had seen information about hate groups.[2] Worse, your daughter could be unwittingly lured into an on-line relationship with someone who could harm her. Increasingly, reports are surfacing about children who make on-line "buddies," and are then lured into meeting their new friends. But these friends turn out to be child molesters or adults who take advantage of children and teens. "Child exploitation on the Internet is one of the fastest-growing forms of exploitation," says Dr. Daniel Broughton, chair of the National Center for Missing and Exploited Children.

The Current TV Ratings Box Definitions

In 1997, the TV industry began using these ratings, called the Parental Guidelines.

Content Labels

V	Violence
S	Sexual situations
L	Coarse or crude, indecent language
D	Suggestive dialogue (usually means talk about sex)
FV	Fantasy violence
TV Y	All children
TV Y7	Directed to Older Children (age seven or above)
TV T7 FV	Directed to Older Children—Fantasy Violence (a kids' show but may feature violence)
TV G	General Audience (usually appropriate for all ages)
TV PG	Parental Guidance Suggested (may have moderate violence, some sexual situations, infrequent coarse language, or some suggestive dialogue)
TV 14	Parents Strongly Cautioned (may have intense violence; intense sexual situations; strong, coarse language; or intensely suggestive dialogue)
TV MA	Mature Audience Only (unsuitable for children under 17)

Set firm safety rules around use of the Internet in your home. You can program your computer to allow your child access to only certain sites, such as kids' sites. Tell your daughter that she should never give out personal information, such as her name, password, address, phone number, or even her school. Instruct your daughter to report to you any instances where she receives or reads offensive or threatening communications, and then report these abuses to your Internet service provider. Be aware that even kids' chat rooms can get badly out of hand. Finally, explain to your daughter that the Internet is not much different than being out in public. She should be wary of strangers. You can double-check your daughter's Internet practices by typing her name or nickname on a search engine to see if it reveals sites or message boards she has visited. But the best way is to be physically present when your daughter is on-line. Or, enter a kids' or teen chat room yourself and get an idea about what kinds of conversations go on. Explain to your daughter that crude or offensive language is no more acceptable on-line than it is in regular conversation. If your daughter is spending inordinate amounts of time on-line, it would be good to ask yourself and her why this is occurring. Is it because your relationship is not as good as it could be? Or because your daughter feels she has no friends other than her on-line buddies? If either of these situations is accurate, turn off the computer and work on the relationship issues.

Warning Signs that Your Child May Be Using the Internet Inappropriately

- Compulsion to use on-line services during much of free time and evening hours
- Participation in chat rooms meant for adults
- Downloading many files
- Receiving phone calls at home from strangers
- Wanting to meet people she has met on-line

Why Some Girls Are at Risk

"My dad drinks too much sometimes and gets wild. He beats us and beats my mom. I feel really bad, and I just go hide in my room."
—Nina, age fourteen

Poverty and social inequities place some girls in environments where they are more at risk of becoming victims of violence or witnessing violence. But, sadly, events such as the Columbine shootings show us that no family is immune to the threat of violence.

Guns are very accessible, even to young people. Some children and teenagers even say that they don't think they'll live to an old age because of the pervasive threat of gun violence. Many gun owners are careless about how they store their weapons. According to one survey, at least 21 percent of gun owners kept at least one gun loaded and in an unlocked setting.[3]

Ask the parents of your daughter's friends if they have a gun in their home. If so, have they taken measures to safeguard it? Your daughter should know that she should call you immediately if she sees a gun at another person's home.

Nationwide, 4.4 percent of students say they have missed a day of school due to fears that they are unsafe at school or getting to and from school.[4] Encourage your daughter to tell you if she is afraid in any environment. If she is worried about getting to and from school, talk to the principal about options to help her. Alert the local police when there are problem streets that school children must traverse. Organize a neighborhood service in which adults take turns walking a group of children to and from school.

Diane lives in a poor neighborhood and worries constantly about her daughter, Jennifer, who is ten. "She has been pretty traumatized by boys. She is always being called names; always being hit and kicked. I can usually tell when this is happening because she starts saying she wants to stay home from school. I start asking more questions than usual. I tell her that it is not okay to be treated like that and that she must say something to someone when it happens."

"I get stressed out thinking about gangs. I'm always looking over my shoulder . . . it's scary."

—Sophia, thirteen (Girls Inc.)

While boys are more often the victims and perpetrators of violence, girls—black girls in particular—are more often witness to violent crimes and exhibit more symptoms of post-traumatic stress disorder.[5] Children who witness violence will often act aggressively with others.[6] Girls are even becoming more likely to commit acts of violence. Female media heroes who can whip the bad guys create the image for girls that it's okay to be tough and physically aggressive.

Your daughter needs to understand the difference in being assertive and able to defend herself physically and being an instigator of physical violence. Violence is not normal behavior. It is unacceptable behavior. Girls who live in gang-infested neighborhoods may be especially vulnerable to joining gangs and embracing the ethic of violence. Your daughter needs to know that gangs are dead-end traps. She should avoid gangs at all costs, because once she joins, it is very hard to break free of a gang.

Parents need to monitor their own behavior. If there is violence in your marriage, understand that you or your spouse are not the only victims. Your daughter is learning by example. Witnessing violence at home, school, or in the neighborhood is strongly correlated to children behaving violently with others.[7] Parents' failure to monitor their children's exposure to violence and media exposure are other factors in children becoming violent. Watch how you control your temper.

Sexual Abuse

A woman is raped in America once every two minutes— one of the highest rates in the world. Young women are especially likely to fall victim to rape, with most victims between eleven and seventeen years old. Rape can be committed by an acquaintance or a stranger. Teach your daughter that *it is impossible to know by looking at someone if he is a rapist*. There are clues that a person might be capable of rape, however. Men who rape are often substance abusers, treat women poorly, think women ask for rape, read pornography, and were sexually active at a young age.

Some men feel they have the right to have sex with a woman whenever they want it. In fact, the majority of women who are raped know their perpetrator. Date rape occurs most often to high school seniors or college freshmen. Your daughter needs to know that saying "no" forcefully and repeatedly should stop unwanted advances. Any resistance from her date should cause your daughter to leave the room immediately.

You can help your daughter by teaching her that rape occurs frequently in this country and that she must use wise judgment to protect herself. The fear of rape should not overcome your daughter or prevent her from having a social life. But she should also practice basic safety measures to minimize her risk. A typical acquaintance-rape scenario involves a party with peers in which a girl drinks or uses drugs and loses her ability to protect herself and think wisely. More than half of girls who are raped by someone they know were using drugs or alcohol before the attack.[8]

Clues that May Mean a Man Is Capable of Rape

- Bossy and controlling
- Becomes easily jealous of time girl spends with others
- Tries to dictate what girl does, wears, and how she spends her time, even what to think
- Treats women poorly, saying degrading things
- Acts superior to women
- Drinks or uses drugs
- Is physically violent
- Puts pressure on girl to have sex
- Has a terrible temper

Women who are raped can suffer a wide range of health consequences. They can experience post-traumatic stress disorder. They often fear their attacker will find them again. They have suicidal thoughts. Some may feel guilty about the assault and blame themselves. Other women will begin using alcohol or drugs. Sexual abuse has emerged as a major reason why some girls have sex too early or become pregnant. Tracy told her stepmother, Barrie, that she had been sexually abused by her mother's boyfriend a few years earlier, before she came to live with her father and Barrie. "She disclosed this to me when she had lived with us for about one year. She told me that when her mother would go out, (the boyfriend) would touch her private parts. This has caused a lot of problems for her. She has no self-confidence and is very self-conscious."

It's important that a woman who is raped seek immediate help, preferably at a rape crisis treatment center. First go to the nearest medical center. Once there, ask if there is a rape crisis center in your community. Counselors are available who will help a victim of rape through the medical exam and questioning by law enforcement authorities and the psychological trauma of the experience. A rape victim should receive medication to prevent sexually transmitted diseases and pregnancy.

"We put Marissa in a martial arts class so she will be able to defend herself if the situation ever arises. I tell her if anyone tries to take her that she must kick and scream and flail her arms," says Terry, whose daughter, now fourteen, was sexually abused at age six. Many girls benefit from classes in self-defense. These classes often help girls become aware of dangerous situations and give them techniques to respond with if attacked. Fighting an attacker is a last resort, however. The biggest benefit from self-defense instruction is that it may help make your daughter more aware of her surroundings and minimize her risks while giving her confidence that she can protect herself.

Information You Can Give Your Daughter for Protection Against Rape and Assault

- Always walk with other people.
- Walk quickly, purposefully, and with an air of confidence.
- Be aware of your surroundings. Before you leave a building or a car, look around and see how well-lit the area is. Are other people around? What is the most direct route to take to your destination?
- Always keep car and house doors and windows locked.
- Don't associate with strangers; even ones you've met an hour or two ago and have had a conversation with. Never leave a party with someone you've just met that evening.
- Don't accept drinks from anyone you don't know. Drinks can be laced with drugs that cause a woman to become unconscious and allow an attack.
- Don't use drugs and alcohol.

Dating Violence

The estimates for how often dating violence occurs range widely. But it is clear from numerous surveys of teens that dating violence happens a lot. Your daughter should understand that violence, in any form, has no place in dating. It's important for adolescents to learn this because patterns of dating in the teen years often carry over into adult life. Beating is the major cause of physical injury to women.

"While society is becoming more aware of domestic violence involving adults, the issue of dating violence among younger adults and adolescents has not received sufficient attention."

—The Journal of the American Medical
Women's Association

Dating violence can include verbal, physical, or sexual violence. While girls are more likely to suffer severe injuries at the
hands of boys, girls themselves are sometimes perpetrators of
violence and tend to inflict minor physical injuries on others.
Girls who assault others are more likely to have been victims of
assault themselves in a dating relationship.[9]

Dating violence often occurs on the part of the male partner
because of anger or the desire to control a girl. Violence can also
occur during arguments over jealousy, sex, friends, and parents.[10]
Violence can even occur because kids believe it is acceptable
behavior. A girl who is pregnant is at higher-than-normal risk of
being physically abused by a male partner.

Typically, teenagers misinterpret dating violence as signs of
love and commitment. For this reason, girls may be unwilling to
leave the relationship.[11] Girls may express love for their abusers
and defend their actions. They may minimize or deny the abuse
or blame themselves for bringing it on. They may be too embarrassed to tell anyone. Some girls keep abuse a secret because they
don't want their parents to break up the relationship or they are
afraid of losing their freedom. Sometimes, girls are afraid to leave
an abusive relationship for fear that the spurned partner will come
after her to hurt or kill her.

Your daughter needs to know that love should never be abusive. No one has the right to hurt her, terrorize her, or make her
afraid. You have to be very attuned to your daughter to pick up on
signs that she may be involved in an abusive relationship. In one
study, only 4 percent of girls told an authority figure that they were
in an abusive relationship.[12] Very few teenagers are capable of extri-
cating themselves from this frightening situation and your daughter
will need your help. Some of the clues to look for include:

- Does your daughter's boyfriend appear to prevent her from talking
  to or being with other friends?

- Does there seem to be a high level of jealousy in the relationship?
- Does the boyfriend call a lot, appearing to check up on your daughter?
- Does your daughter comment that her boyfriend likes her to only wear certain styles of clothes or talk to certain friends? Does he appear to be dictating her behavior in any other ways or intimidating her?
- Does your daughter appear worried about the relationship?
- Does your daughter complain about vague stomachaches, headaches, or other pain?

Confront your daughter gently about your worries. Instead of criticizing her boyfriend, talk to her about how great she is and how she deserves to be treated well. Encourage her to talk to a counselor or therapist. Be patient and supportive. Acknowledge her feelings but tell her yours, too, such as "I'm afraid for you." Try to get your daughter to agree to take small steps, such as limiting the places in which she can see her boyfriend to obviously safe areas. Remind her that you will always pick her up if she calls you—no matter what the circumstances. Buy her a cellular telephone or prepaid phone card. Tell other people who are around your daughter, such as teachers, neighbors, or friends, that you are afraid for your daughter and to please watch out for her safety. In some cases, it may be necessary for both your daughter's sake and for the sake of other girls who may become victims of violence to report a man's behavior to authorities.

Sexual Harassment

Rhonda, fourteen, says sexual harassment is a common part of middle school. "It's a big deal to me. A girl in one of my classes has bigger breasts than most of us. A boy went up and pulled the back of her bra and broke it. Now everyone is pulling each other's bras. My advice is, don't wear a bra unless you need one."

Sexual harassment is a pervasive part of American society. About 70 percent of female students have reported sexual harassment at school.[13] And one-quarter of those girls said the harassment came from adults, including teachers. Harassment can start in elementary school.[14] No groups are immune from this socially ingrained practice, although Hispanic girls report more incidents of sexual insults than do members of other racial or ethnic groups. Sexual harassment is so entrenched that it has only been recently that women have spoken out against the abuse and laws have been enacted to prevent it.

Sexual harassment has four elements: It is sexual in nature, unwelcome, repetitive, and behavior that most people would consider offensive. It can include sexual comments, teasing, gestures, or jokes; being flashed, touched, brushed up against, pinched, or hugged. It can involve spreading rumors about a girl's sexuality or being spied on or surreptitiously filmed while changing clothes or in a shower. It can be offensive graffiti, drawings, cartoons, or pornography being shown or distributed in inappropriate places, such as school or work. Sexual harassment is even perpetrated by companies, such as the California surf wear company that once printed the slogan "Destroy All Girls" on its clothing line or the doll designed as a male wrestler who carried a woman's head in his hands.

Trina struggles with what to tell her daughter, Hannah, fifteen, about sexual harassment. Trina is employed in a business with mostly men, and she knows all too well what kinds of things are said. "I probably will tell her to speak up and defend herself, since it is a cowardly act and the perpetrator will likely back off. But if the harassment is done in private I would suggest that she get out of whatever situation she is in and consider reporting it to the proper authority."

Teenagers who work under the supervision of an adult too often experience sexual harassment. One poll of 1,000 teen girls found that 20 percent reported sexual harassment in the workplace. Of those who reported harassment, more than half said it took the form of offensive jokes or conversation or flirtatious comments and unwanted advances from bosses or coworkers. This is a vulnerable situation for a girl because it may be her first job and she could be extremely reluctant to stand up to the boss. The harassment can even take the form of bribes, such as "go out on a date with me and I'll give you a raise."

Part of your daughter's preparation for her first job should include a discussion with you on her right to a respectful and safe workplace. It doesn't matter if she's the CEO or earning minimum wage. She needs to know that there are appropriate channels—even specific paperwork—that allows her to complain about sexual harassment on the job without losing her job.

> "In seventh grade, a group of boys made up a 'flat chest club.' They put a few of my friends and me in it. We told a teacher so they'd stop talking about it. All the other girls in my class were mad at us for getting the guys in trouble. One of them walked up to us and said, 'You're so stupid.'"
>
> —A teen girl, from "Voices of a Generation: Teenage Girls on Sex, School and Self," American Association of University Women, 1999

Girls may worry that they are overreacting because sexual harassment can be communicated in a joking manner. Explain to your daughter that if the behavior makes her feel uncomfortable, afraid, or insulted, it is harassment. Some people may try to excuse sexual harassment by saying something like "boys will be boys." Tell your daughter that such reasoning is not an excuse. Caring boys do not act macho, aggressive, or superior to women. Explain to your daughter that sexual harassment emerges from long-ingrained sexist attitudes that some men still harbor against women. Sexual harassment signals a lack of respect for girls and women. It is not the fault of the woman. Although you may know that, your daughter needs to hear that from you.

> "Someone said that I was a slut. You always try to pretend that what people say about you doesn't affect you, but it does. You slowly start to believe what's being said about you."
>
> —A girl, from "Voices of a Generation: Teenage
> Girls on Sex, School and Self," American
> Association of University Women, 1999

The effects of sexual harassment on a girl are tragic. Since it often occurs at school, it can detract from learning and make a girl fearful and unable to concentrate. It destroys self-image and self-esteem in all but the strongest girls. Dealing effectively with the harasser can help your daughter feel vindicated and in control. Discuss how the situation can be handled. Maybe your daughter need only tell the harasser that his behavior is unacceptable and to stop bothering her. If the abuse continues, seek help from an authority, such as the school principal or a manager where your daughter works. Keep a thorough record of the harassing incidents. Sexual harassment is against the law. You may need to file legal action if the abuse is severe and unrelenting. Remember that serious sexual harassment is too difficult for a child to handle alone. You need to be your daughter's ally and fight the battle with her.

Sexual Harassment in Schools

In May 1999, the U.S. Supreme Court ruled that any school receiving federal money can be sued for sex discrimination by failing to intervene in reported cases of sexual harassment of students. Writing for the majority, Justice Sandra Day O'Connor said that student-on-student sexual harassment can impede a child's ability to learn. What this tells children is that adults are supposed to watch out for them at school. Don't be afraid to be a forceful advocate for your daughter and demand a respectful environment in which she can learn. This is the action that Jacqueline took when her eleven-year-old daughter was sexually harassed at school. "First I went to bat for her and talked to the school and the involved parties. She and I came up with strategies for the future. The school suggested she walk away from the situation. I told them that was fine, but it was not her responsibility to put an end to the situation, nor should she always have to stop what she is doing to get away from the harassment. Boys need to learn that their behavior is not okay. It is the school's responsibility to make school environments safe."

Be sure your daughter doesn't switch sides and become a harasser. One of the consequences of empowering girls is that some girls will misuse their empowerment and will perpetrate the same kinds of abuses on males as males have on them. In some schools, these girls are even called names like "stalker chicks." They harass boys, vandalize their lockers or cars, call them on the telephone or E-mail them relentlessly, or even slap or push boys. This is as equally unacceptable as any harassment perpetrated by males upon females.

A policy of zero tolerance of violence and any form of abuse will not only make your daughter's life easier, it will give her confidence and a greater sense of self-worth. Consider that one of your family values should be the right of every person to be treated with respect and dignity. A girl who lives by this value will reap the benefits in each and every relationship.

Questions to Ask Your Doctor

- My daughter was the victim of severe harassment for part of a school year. She is now having chronic nightmares. Is this post-traumatic stress syndrome?
- We keep a gun in the house for personal safety. Where should we put it and what should we tell our children about our keeping a gun?
- My husband occasionally strikes me when he is angry or upset, and my daughter has witnessed these incidents. Will this have any harmful effects on her?
- At what age should I allow my child to begin watching shows that aren't just "children's shows"?
- My child acts very aggressively and has even slapped and shoved other girls. What does this mean, and how can I help her overcome this aggressive behavior?

Resources

- *FamilyPC* magazine has a web site to help parents check out the content of popular computer games at www.familypc.com.
- You can identify violent computer games by checking the box for a rating from the Entertainment Software Rating Board at ww.esrb.org.
- The Lion & Lamb Project is an organization that encourages parents to protest violence in children's entertainment. It is located at www.lionlamb.org.
- The National Institute on Media and the Family rates video and computer games and provides information on the effects of media exposure. It can be found at www.mediaandthefamily.org.
- Parents can obtain a free booklet on talking with kids about violence by calling 800-CHILD44 or on the web at www.talkingwithkids.org.

- The National Domestic Violence Hotline is open twenty-four hours a day and can provide counseling and information regarding dating violence. Call 800-799-7233.
- Women who have experienced crime can obtain information and resources from the National Organization for Victim Assistance at 888-TRY-NOVA.
- The National Organization for Women's Legal Defense and Action Kit has a booklet called *Sexual Harassment in the Schools* that offers information and guidance. It can be obtained for $5 from NOW Legal Defense Fund, 99 Hudson Street, New York, NY 10013.
- A helpful book for women to prevent victimization is *A Woman's Guide to Personal Safety*, by Janee Harteau and Holly Keegel (Fairview Press, 1998).
- Information on preventing school violence can be obtained from the Center for the Prevention of School Violence at 800-299-6054.
- The Institute for Mental Health Initiatives' Channeling Children's Anger report has tips to help parents. Call 202-467-2285.
- The National Foundation Collaborative on Violence Prevention offers information and resources. Call 202-393-7731 or visit www.usakids.org.
- The Pacific Center for Violence Prevention is a good source for information on prevention. Call 415-285-1793 or visit www.pcvp.org.
- *Talking With Your Child About a Troubled World*, by Lynne S. Dumas (Ballentine Books, 1992), is a helpful book for parents who aren't sure how to begin a conversation with their child.
- A good guide on understanding the TV rating system and how the V-Chip works can be ordered from the Center for Media Education and the Kaiser Family Foundation. It's entitled *Parent's Guide to the TV Ratings and V-Chip*. Call 800-656-4533 (publication #1491) or check out the V-Chip Education Project web site at www.vchipeducation.org.

- Girls who encounter violence frequently in their communities will benefit from this overall health guide, *Finding Our Way: The Teen Girls' Survival Guide*, by Allison Abner and Linda Villarosa (Harper-Perennial, 1995). It has a detailed section on coping with unsafe environments.
- *The Date Rape Prevention Book: The Essential Guide for Girls & Women*, by crime prevention specialist Scott Lindquist (Source-books, Inc., 2000), is a straightforward advice book that will inform without frightening teenagers.

CHAPTER 16

Education: The Sky's the Limit

"Girls should be told that what they say matters and they are important. All people who want to learn should be in certain classes and
the people who don't take school seriously should be in other
classes so the people who want to learn can learn."
—Darla, age fourteen, from the American
Associate of University Women's *Voices of a
New Generation* report, 1999

IT MAY seem odd to have a chapter on education in a book
about health. What does health have to do with education?
Although the ties to health and education are indirect, they are
tightly linked. Girls who obtain a good education are much more

likely to practice healthy habits and be vigilant about health over their lifespan. A quality education not only teaches your daughter about disease, nutrition, fitness, and other health topics, it provides her with the thinking skills, self-esteem, determination, and pride to protect her most cherished asset: her health.

As the parent of a girl, you must be more proactive about your daughter's education and plans for her future than you would with a son. Women have made progress in attaining economic and career equality with men, but there is still ground to make up. Think of it this way: Despite the fact that your daughter may have graduated from her college class sharing a 4.0 grade point average with a boy, discrimination and pay inequality may make it seem as if she scored perhaps a 3.7. Like members of minority groups, girls today generally still have to work harder and be more assertive to obtain the educational and career rewards accessible to bright boys. Betsy and Ray have made it clear to their daughter, Rachel, sixteen, that she needs a good education, even if she gets married and has the "lots of kids" that she often talks about. "We always discuss her education with her and how important it is—especially since she is a woman. She knows that post–high school education is essential. Without that, it's tough."

A girl who aims high in school reaps more than good grades and potential career rewards. She has more reasons to avoid the risk-taking behavior that undermines good school performance, such as substance abuse. Lillian explains that her daughter, Missy, fifteen, is unaffected by pressures to smoke or use alcohol or drugs, saying: "She's pretty interested in going on to a great school, and looks at most things from that perspective."

Gender Stereotyping in Education

In the early 1990s, educators were stung by criticism that they favored male students, calling on boys more often and setting

More Years in School Equals Better Health

In almost every measure of health, highly educated women show better results and greater success at accessing preventive health services. This chart shows the percentage of adult women who reported having a mammogram.

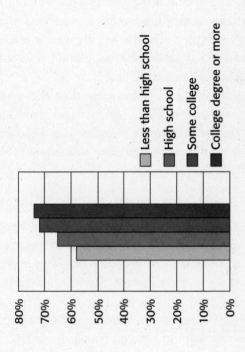

Source: Centers for Disease Control and Prevention, Sept. 14, 1990.

higher standards for them.[1] Tonya, a parent who spends many hours volunteering in her daughter's middle school, says she has witnessed this phenomenon firsthand. "The teacher calls on the boys more and expects more of them," Tonya says, "particularly in science." While surveys tell us that teachers are becoming more aware of the need to call on boys and girls equally, they still may not provide girls with as much direct feedback or criticism as boys for fear of hurting girls' feelings.[2] This further disadvantages girls because they need to learn to respond to criticism. But perhaps the biggest area where girls are not reaching high enough, and are not walking on equal ground with boys, is in studies of math, science, and technology.

It's been known for some time that girls tend to achieve lower scores than boys in science and math. That gap is narrowing. But when it comes to technology—the defining industry of the new millenium—girls are still falling short. Consider these sobering facts:

- Girls are more likely to take clerical and data entry classes.
- Girls have fewer female role models in computer games and educational software. One study of computer games with gender-identifiable characters found only 12 percent were female, and many of these characters represented traditional roles, such as mother or princess.
- Girls use computers less often outside of school.
- Computer use between boys and girls tends to be about equal until age twelve, when boys begin to spend more time on computers.
- Computer games for girls make up less than 5 percent of the billion-dollar market.
- Only 17 percent of high school students taking Advanced Placement tests in computer science are girls.

This is an inventory to assess your school's work on gender equity. Does your school have:

- Policies that make gender issues a priority?
- Support for girls of all races, languages, negotiating strategies, and physical abilities?
- Adults with whom girls can talk about issues such as sexuality, birth control, and family and peer pressures?
- Support in the school and the district for adults who mentor girls?
- Equitable athletic programs?
- A sexual harassment policy?
- Data that show student achievement by gender?
- Professional development to help teachers make their classrooms more equitable?
- Curricula and teaching approaches that encourage girls and boys to try out a range of roles in the process of identity development?
- Adults and programs offering leadership opportunities to girls of diverse cultures who use a range of negotiating strategies?
- Girls, parents, and school staff involved in assessing the school experience for girls and in shaping reform?
- Forums for dialogue across the various constituencies of the school community?

Source: American Association of University Women Educational Foundation.

In today's society, girls need a comfort level with science, math, and technology. They need to be confident of their ability to handle money and finance.

Computers

You can help your daughter by educating yourself about computers if you don't already have some basic knowledge. If you don't have a home computer, check your local library or school to find out if you can have free or low-cost access. If you can afford it, there are many computer education businesses that have classes for adults and children. Check into computer summer camps, too.

It's imperative today that children learn typing, or keyboard, skills well before high school. It's okay to start with a child as young as eight. Teach your daughter some fundamentals, such as the concept that the right hand reaches for the keys on the right side of the keyboard and the left hand reaches for the left keys. By age ten, your daughter can begin to learn which fingers stroke certain keys. Many schools have courses in keyboarding for children. Or you can purchase a good learn-to-type computer program. If you don't have a home computer, talk to your daughter's teacher about how much keyboarding instruction she'll receive in school.

Consider starting a girls' computer club. Your daughter and her friends can build their own home page, for instance, with some guidance from you. Maybe a local computer or software company or store will sponsor you. You can even plan field trips to learn more about computers. Look for good web sites for girls that will engage them. Be aware that when girls do use computers, however, they may unknowingly become the target of marketers who do more to advance gender stereotyping than break it. Girls are often targeted for surveys that reveal their likes and dislikes. These surveys are then sold to marketers who advertise to girls. Instruct your daughter to ignore solicitations for her opinions.

Finance

Finance is another skill that is frequently overlooked in girls' education. One study found that parents teach boys and girls about money much differently. Boys typically learn a lot more about money and are given more responsibility with money. They are encouraged to appreciate and earn money. Many girls, meanwhile, tend to view money as "tainted" and say they would feel guilty if they earned a lot of money.

Avoiding Injuries from Computer Use

Just like adults, children who use a computer a lot can develop repetitive stress injuries. Here are some tips that will help your daughter develop healthy computer habits.

- Teach your daughter the warning signs of repetitive stress injuries, such as tingling in the hands or wrists, pain, shoulder or upper back stiffness or soreness. Your daughter should tell you immediately if she suffers from any of these symptoms.
- Make sure the equipment your child uses is appropriate for her size. Children need chairs that fit to their desks. The computer monitor should be directly in front of the child with the top of the screen at eye level. The keyboard and mouse should be low enough to allow the child to relax her shoulders.
- Tell your child to take frequent breaks from computer use. Just as television viewing allows for long periods of sedentary behavior, so does the computer. Set a time limit for computer use, such as one hour.
- Teach your daughter good posture. This includes not resting her wrists on the desk or keyboard while typing or using the mouse.

Source: Deborah Quilter, www.rsihelp.com/children.html. Quilter is also the author of *The Repetitive Strain Injury Recovery Book* (Walker, 1998).

Teach your daughter how to handle money by giving her an allowance. Explain to her that the ATM at the bank doesn't just give away money. Tell her how you earn the money, deposit it at the bank, and carefully withdraw it when needed. Eventually, introduce her to the idea of saving and investing. Let her help you sort through bills and explain how you handle money. Teenagers can learn to read the stock market listings in the newspaper business pages. Don't allow yourself to support your daughter financially any longer than you would support your son.

Math

Women who take more than two college math courses typically earn as much as men. But you need to start young.[4] Don't let her wiggle out of algebra when it first becomes optional (usually about eighth grade). And don't allow her (or yourself) to panic if math occasionally becomes a struggle. Let her know that it's natural for all math students to become lost and confused at times. It's very important for your daughter to understand that she must ask for help from the teacher when she doesn't understand something. Some girls are too shy or embarrassed to speak up when they are confused. This is an unfortunate behavior that you should discourage.

Don't buy into the idea that boys are naturally better at math than girls and girls will inevitably struggle. Science hasn't resolved the debate over whether a certain gender is born with more ability in a particular skill. Besides, it doesn't matter. All kids who intend to have successful careers need to have good math skills—whether it comes naturally or not.[5]

Science

It's no surprise that women make up less than one-third of the science labor force and only 8 percent of engineers.[6] Science is a profession that still holds a certain mystique over nonscientists. It can be very easy for your daughter to become intimidated with the idea of a career in science, even if she loves science classes. A good way to help her overcome this fear of the unknown is to help her meet some women scientists. (For example, volunteer to work at her school's career day and then find and invite some female scientists.) Or you could locate summer science camps and inquire about which ones work especially hard to help girls envision careers in science. Books and web sites about women in science are also wonderful, and there are several to choose from (see Resources). Reading about the real lives (including marriages) of women scientists helps greatly to demystify the profession.

Jean and Terry often talk to their daughters, Mindi and Nicole, about science, even though both girls prefer, and do better, in language arts. "I think they are naturally more talented in the arts, although their grasp of scientific things is quite broad. Terry is a scientist and has explained things to them since they were very small," says Jean. This is good advice. If your daughter shies away from math and science, look for opportunities to interpret it and show her how it applies to real life (such as how you need to balance your checkbook or how you go about fixing an appliance). The most important predictor of a career in science is the number of elective science courses girls take in high school. Encourage your daughter to take at least a few basic science courses in high school, even if she is uninterested in science. If your daughter does show a preference for science, plan how she can make the most of middle school and high school science course offerings.[7]

Achievement

"Achievement is not about what you've done, but what you've gained from your experience."

—Lynn Hill, rock climber, from *A Girl's Book of Wisdom*, edited by Catherine Dee (Little, Brown, 1990)

Jessica is ten and exuberant about her future. "The girls in my class are sooooo much smarter than the boys. The teachers know we're smarter, but they just won't admit it in front of the boys." Would that Jessica could maintain that boastful confidence! But history tells us that most girls don't. Girls tend to do better in school through third grade. Then the balance tips in favor of boys. This appears to occur for several reasons: Teachers give boys more attention, feedback, and praise; parents demand more of boys; and girls' self-esteem declines as they begin to realize that society places more value on how they look than on what they achieve.[8]

Girls seem to easily lose their confidence in their academic abilities. Around fourth grade, boys tend to overestimate their school performance and attribute failure to bad luck, the difficulty of the task, or not trying hard enough. Girls tend to underestimate their performance and attribute school failures to their own low ability.[9] The pattern tends to show up in subsequent years and can even augment other insecurities. By seventh grade, girls who underestimate their school abilities often show signs of anxiety and depression.

> "Believing that one is competent or capable of handling a particular task can be highly motivating, even when it is not true."
>
> —David A. Cole, psychologist, University of Notre Dame

You can have an impact on your daughter's education simply through your support and attitude. Try not to scold or nag your daughter about schoolwork. Instead, look for opportunities to praise her performance. Beginning in the early grades, hang well-done work on the refrigerator or family bulletin board. Let your daughter know that you think she is smart and expect her to do very well. Studies show that children's intrinsic motivation to do well in school is directly influenced by their parents' encouragement.[10]

Concentrate on praising your daughter for her effort, as opposed to her ability or intelligence.[11] Praise for effort tends to encourage a love of learning while praise for ability tends to emphasize performance, such as grades.

**Parents' Tips for Encouraging
High-Achieving School Performance**

- "We teach her that her heart is just as important as her mind."
- "I expect her to try her hardest. If that equates to a C, that's okay as long as it's the best she can do."
- "I'm very involved in her education. I've been a room mom. I'm always a classroom helper, and I make it a point to get to know the other children in the class."
- "We don't allow TV on Monday through Thursday nights, and I sit with my three children while they do their homework."
- "I go to the opportunities at school to meet the teachers and contact them if I see any issues that are overwhelming her."
- "I try to let her handle most things first, but if she asks for our intervention or help we do so."
- "We discuss every paper and every grade and why it was what it was; whether the teacher was unfair; what she could have done better."

Keep in mind that studies universally show that a family that is close, connected, and caring gets better school performances from their children. Your daughter needs to know that you are available to her when she needs you (not necessarily only when it's convenient for you). As children get older, parental involvement in education tends to fall off dramatically.[12] Only about half of all high school parents say they are involved at school in some way, such as the PTA, volunteer work, or helping at school. Begin each school year with a personal commitment to select at least one way to be involved in your daughter's school. Sherrice, who has two girls, has the right attitude: "I strongly feel that an active parent has an active child. If your child sees that you are interested in her education, it makes all the difference in the world. If you're not involved, why should she be involved or care?"

All-Girls Education

Some parents feel their daughters will do best in an all-girls school. There is good data to support this belief.[13] All-girls schools are committed to creating learning environments in which girls excel. They study and understand what it takes for girls to reach their highest potential. In all-girls schools there are no worries that girls will get second-class status. Each student in an all-girls school is expected to participate and be successful. This often leads students to take more risks, develop more confidence and independence, and feel freer to express themselves. The distraction of boys is absent.

Statistics point out some favorable aspects to all-girls education. In all-girls schools, 80 percent of girls take four years of math and science compared with two years for most girls in coed schools. All-girls schools have produced many social and political leaders. One-third of the female board members of Fortune 1,000 companies went to all-girls schools. There is no good evidence, however, that girls in all-girls school do better in an overall sense.[14] Nevertheless, many educators do believe that girls' learning styles differ from boys and that single-sex classes benefit girls.

All-girls schools are typically private and cost a lot of money. But more public schools are starting to offer segregated math and science classes. Ask your school's principal or members of your district school board to analyze the test scores or grades for math, science, and computer science by gender. If girls are falling short of boys, you have a good case for arguing that optional, segregated classes be offered.

Careers

"A girl is watching. What is she learning?"

–Theme from the Ms. Foundation Take Our
Daughters to Work Day

Do you ever wonder what your daughter's life will be like when she is an adult?[15] Here is a scenario that is quite realistic: A girl in the next generation will face aggressive and competitive job markets, the need to earn her own income working outside the home, the need to work outside the home for most of her life, the strong possibility of experiencing conflicts between children, home, and careers, the strong possibility of being sexually harassed on the job, the possibility that she will make more money than her husband, and that she may spend some sizable portion of her career as her home's sole breadwinner.

In other words, there are few indications that your daughter will have it easy (although gains women have made in the workplace and more equality in parenting may ease the burden for help in future generations). Your daughter needs your help and support in developing a plan—a dream—to pursue in adulthood. Mother-daughter relationships, in particular, contribute greatly to girls' career choices.

So what can you do? Here are some suggestions:

- Look for community programs, summer camps, and contests that foster your daughter's interest in math, science, and technology.
- Participate in Take Our Daughters to Work Day. Mothers are especially useful role models because they demonstrate how they juggle their various roles of wife, mother, and employee. Be honest about the hardships involved in the working world. Girls want, and can handle, the truth. Don't hold your daughter to expectations of perfection in either her education or career. As experts from the

Ms. Foundation say : "... being a 'perfect girl' is still a strong and often debilitating theme in girls' lives."[16]

• Encourage your daughter to start her own mini-business—babysitting, dog walking, making jewelry or crafts, washing cars, mowing lawns. When my daughters and a friend across the street decided to open a cookie and lemonade stand one hot summer day, I overcame my initial dread and got behind them. Four hours later, they were wallowing in $15 cash and were proud of their profit-enhancing creation of a drive-through cookie and lemonade stand. (They waved the neighbors' cars down as they came around the corner.)

"Although true equality for women has not yet arrived in our nation, your daughters can pass through doors that women never dared to dream of entering only a generation ago."

—Dr. Sylvia Rimm, *See Jane Win*

If you want to know how girls become successful women, what better way than to ask 1,000 of them. That is what Dr. Sylvia Rimm, a researcher at Case Western Reserve University School of Medicine, did. With the help of her two grown daughters, both of whom are medical professionals, Rimm asked successful women in all types of careers—medicine, technology, education, mental health, journalism, and other areas—about the factors, conditions, and actions that influenced their careers. Rimm's results, published in the book *See Jane Win*, are a treasure trove of sound advice on how you can help your daughter succeed.

It's imperative that both parents set high expectations for their daughters. Rimm found that about 70 percent of women said they felt both their father and mother had encouraged them to reach high. Many of the successful women were smart and got good grades in school. And many had experienced success already, such as by having a work of art displayed or by winning a competition. But what may be more important, says Rimm, is that these women learned to embrace a solid work ethic and fought hard to achieve their goals. Successful women were raised to be highly motivated, hardworking, and independent.

Be aware of how you communicate about your daughter and to her, Rimm says. Be careful in your choice of words. "You played that song so well" is a much different message than "You look so pretty today." Reinforce the qualities that you want your daughter to have. Avoid using superlatives, such as calling your daughter the "smartest" or "perfect."

If you have not had a career, encourage your daughter to find a mentor who can guide her in technical aspects of career development. Having a mentor is inspiring and, usually, imperative in the development of a professional career. This can be a teacher, principal, counselor, coach, or co-worker. Help your daughter find an adult with whom she connects. You, however, are still your daughter's best source of encouragement, love, and support.

Rimm's findings are too numerous to summarize, but here are some of her major observations about what girls need to succeed (based on a poll of 1,000 successful career women).

1. Set high educational goals for your daughters, such as college and beyond. Discuss careers with them.
2. Allow your daughter to feel some pressure. She needs this to build resilience. On the other hand, don't set unrealistically high expectations. If your daughter shows signs of too much pressure, help her manage her time better.
3. Let your daughter know that you think she is intelligent.
4. Value work; including your own work. Teach her to love accomplishment.
5. Being shy or kind won't necessarily interfere with a good career. Assertiveness can be learned. But misbehavior in your daughter, such as being manipulative or rude, should be addressed and corrected.

6. Many successful women attended public schools, although there may be some advantages to parochial, private, or independent schools. If finances are limited, high school may be a more important time to choose a school that requires tuition.

7. Encourage your daughter to develop math and science skills. Make reading a high priority. Read to and with your daughter.

8. Set aside your own fears about math and encourage your daughter. She will have more career choices if she conquers advanced math. It's worthwhile even if she gets lower grades in math than in other subjects.

9. If your daughter is not challenged academically, ask for her to be moved ahead or skipped a grade.

10. Make room for extracurricular activities, such as music, art, Girl Scouts, band, drama, religion or sports. Girls will learn to manage busy schedules. Make sure, however, that your daughter has downtime for her to fill with her own imagination and self-entertainment.

11. Persuade your daughter that competition is healthy and that it's okay to be competitive. Winning all the time is not possible. It's important to experience losing, too. Winning builds confidence while losing builds character.

12. Travel as a family and allow your daughter to travel independently when she's old enough. Mother-daughter and father-daughter trips are also enriching.

13. Try to downplay the importance of being socially popular with peers. Encourage your daughter to avoid negative friends and encourage her to value independence from her peers. Tell your daughter that everyone, even adults, is lonely sometimes. Don't allow your daughter's active social life with friends to interfere or overshadow private family time.

14. Keep tales of your own use of alcohol, tobacco, or drugs to a minimum and don't glorify it. Make it clear that you expect that she will not smoke, drink, or use drugs.

15. Remind your daughter that you are an ally, not an enemy. Don't accept rebellion. Let your daughter have some freedom with limits. If she misbehaves, don't take away positive activities as punishments.

16. Birth order is not a major factor in success. Don't baby the youngest daughter and don't label your children as the "smart one" or the "athletic one." Your daughters can be many things without being the "most" or "best."

17. Mothers, know that your daughters are watching you. If you want to advance your career or return to school, do it. They will see you as courageous and competent and will benefit even more than if you stay at home.

18. Expect ups and downs in your daughter's life. Setbacks are not permanent, so don't get overly upset. Don't overprotect your daughter. Let her know that she will survive.

19. Teach your daughter to look for careers that challenge her, allow her to contribute of herself, and are creative.

20. Explain the transition in life that occurs when career women become mothers. Encourage daughters, if they plan to marry and have children, to choose partners who will be supportive of their careers and who will co-parent equally.

Working

Many girls benefit from taking on occasional jobs like baby-sitting or pet-sitting. This is a great idea. It teaches girls responsibility and how to interact with a psuedo-employer (the neighbor). Your daughter will also experience the feeling of having her own hard-earned money in her pocket. She may have different feelings about how much money she saves or spends when it's money she has earned.

But what happens after she tires of baby-sitting or wants to earn more money? Many parents struggle with whether or not to allow or encourage their high school–aged children to work at regular jobs. A job can be a wonderful experience. And, for teens whose families cannot easily afford college, part-time or summer jobs during the high school years may be a necessity. But there are some things that you should consider when contemplating a real job with your daughter.

One of the most important issues to be clear about—before she takes a job—concerns how many hours she should work. Many employed teens find their hours accumulating surreptitiously. Before you know it, they are struggling to keep up with studies and can't get enough sleep. Spending too much time at a job can have a negative impact on your daughter in other ways, too.[17] While working fifteen hours or less can be good, higher workloads can undermine kids' education and health. There is evidence that intensive work *raises* the risk of drug use and smoking and *lowers* educational attainment

Question your daughter about why she wants to work. Many kids work due to pressures to buy the latest clothes, CDs, surfboards, or for money for class trips or the prom. Persuade your daughter not to fall victim to advertising pressures, which are increasingly focused on teen girls, that make her feel she has to have this piece of clothing or that accessory.

If you and your daughter decide a job is okay, help her think of appropriate places to apply for work. Many youth jobs don't really help kids achieve their long-term educational and career goals. If your daughter does want to work, try to steer her toward a job that furthers her educational goals. Counsel your daughter on what she should expect when being hired. This is the time to point out that prospective employers cannot and should not ask certain questions of her during an interview such as: Do you have a boyfriend? or, What size dress do you wear? While it's quite likely your daughter will only be able to find a job paying minimum wage, remind her that women need to be especially conscious about pay. Despite women's gains in the workplace, women in general still only earn about 83 cents to every dollar earned by a man. Finally, make it your business to ensure that your daughter's work environment is safe. Teenagers are injured on the job in the very same ways that adults are. Ask your daughter if her employer has health and safety guidelines or a training program to ensure her safety. Don't allow your daughter to work in high-risk businesses, such as mini-marts or businesses that maintain late evening hours that are the frequent targets of robbers. Above all, keep talking to your daughter about her long-term goals. A part-time, minimum-wage job shouldn't lure her away from the kind of fulfilling career that only comes with higher education.

Questions to Ask Your Doctor

- My daughter works part-time and takes advanced-placement classes at school. She is exhausted all the time. How much sleep does a girl her age require?
- My third grader has trouble reading. Do learning disabilities appear in particular grades and should we have her tested?
- My husband has attention deficit disorder. Does this condition run in families, and how would I know if my daughter has it?
- My daughter has lots of things going on and is under a lot of stress. She complains of constant headaches. Could this be due to the stress?
- At what age should my child have a vision exam with an optometrist or ophthalmologist?
- My daughter is too shy to answer questions in class. Is this a disorder that can be treated? Or would some kind of counseling or intervention help?

Resources

- The Women's College Coalition has programs that benefit girls' education and career development and advice for parents raising girls. Call 202-234-0443 or visit www.academic.org.
- Integrating Gender Equity and Reform is a multi-university project to support gender equity in classrooms. The web site has teacher training materials, program information for girls, and stories about successful women in the sciences. Visit InGEAR at www.coe.uga.edu/ingear.
- Voices of Girls in Science, Mathematics, and Technology is a program to help girls sponsored by the American Association of University Women and other groups. You can find information for girls as well as research on the topic. Call 800-624-9120 or visit www.ael.org/nsf/voices.
- Girl Tech is a company that produces technological products and toys for girls. The web site has lots of activities for girls, including a chat room, stories about successful women, and more. Visit www.girltech.com.
- Many branches of the American Association of University Women operate math, science, and technology programs for girls. Call 800-326-2289 or visit www.aauw.org.
- *Does Jane Compute? Preserving Our Daughters' Place in the Cyber Revolution,* by Roberta Furger (Warner Books, 1998), is a highly rated book to help girls become computer literate.
- *Schoolgirls: Young Women, Self-Esteem and the Confidence Gap*, by Peggy Orenstein, in association with the American Association of University Women (Doubleday, 1994), is a look at girls in two middle schools and how girls change and succumb to social pressures and expectations.
- Operation SMART is a program from Girls Inc. that helps girls explore opportunities and develop skills in math, science, and technology. For more information call 212-509-2000 or visit the

web site at www.girlsinc.org. Girls Inc. also has an Economic Literacy program to encourage girls to learn about managing money.

- *No More Frogs to Kiss: 99 Ways to Give Economic Power to Girls*, by Joline Godfrey (Harper Business, 1995), gives girls activities that can help them develop business skills. The book also gives girls descriptions of role models.

- Advocates for Women in Science, Engineering and Mathematics is a wonderful resource for information on gender equity, advice to parents, and program and product information. Call 503-748-1261 or visit www.awsem.org.

- *Girl Boss: Running the Show Like the Big Chicks*, by Stacy Kravetz and Amy Inouye (Girl Press, 1999), offers tips and advice for girls and descriptions of girls who have launched businesses. The book discusses what it takes to succeed in business.

- A nice web site with information on 20,000 biographies of women can be found at www.undelete.org.

- *Cool Women*, by Dawn Chipman, Mari Florence, and Naomi Wax (Girl Press, 1998), has stories of historic women heroines. It is part of a series of books for girls that includes *Cool Careers for Girls*, by Ceel Pasternak and Linda Thornburg. Also in the series: *Cool Careers for Girls in Computers, Cool Careers for Girls with Animals*, and *Cool Careers for Girls in Sports*.

- *Girls Who Rocked the World*, by Amelie Welden (Beyond Words, 1998), is for girls in grades four through seven and offers biographical sketches of interesting women and asks girls how they, too, can have an impact.

- Women of NASA can be found at www.quest.arc.nasa.gov/women/intro.html. It includes a place where girls can chat with mentors.

- *Girls Seen and Heard: 52 Life Lessons for Our Daughters*, by the Ms. Foundation for Women (Tarcher/Putnam, 1998), has interactive exercises and thoughts that encourage girls to reach their full potential.

- *Women in Science*, by Vivian Gornick (Touchstone Books, 1990), includes vignettes about the real lives of women in the sciences. It's best suited for high school–aged girls.
- A Girl's World is an on-line site for girls ages seven to seventeen that aims to educate and promote girls' independence through interest in science, math, finances, and technology and by encouraging education. It is written largely by girls. Visit www.agirlsworld.com.
- Girls can find many good programs and camps that foster education in the sciences by reading *The Girl Pages*, by Charlotte Milholland (Hyperion, 1998).
- MentorNet is an Internet-based mentoring program for women pursuing careers in science and engineering. It pairs students with a professional in the field. Visit www.mentornet.net.

CHAPTER 17

Smoking: A "Pediatric Disease"

W HEN I STARTED smoking, it was the cool thing to do," says Tina, an eighteen-year-old college student.[1] "I was twelve. Cigarettes were easy to get and fairly cheap. Most of the people in liquor stores would sell to us without hassling us." After five years of daily smoking, however, Tina began to have second thoughts about smoking. "I realized my health was being affected. I had asthma as a child, and it started up again. I was coughing up disgusting things every morning."

After four months of trying and failing, Tina finally quit smoking. In order to accomplish this, however, she had to drop most of her college friends, all of whom were smokers. But Tina is satisfied that she has corrected a serious problem before it got worse. "I have an elderly relative who is sick, and she refuses to quit smoking. I'm glad I'm not going to be like that."

Given the negative examples before them, it is perplexing that teenage girls—particularly white girls—are the people most likely to begin smoking. While smoking has declined among adults—who now generally recognize its serious health consequences—smoking has increased among youths, *particularly girls*. About 40 percent of all white high school girls now smoke and smoking is dramatically increasing in other ethnic groups, such as among Latinas.[2] More girls than boys are smoking by seventh grade, and the gap widens considerably by ninth grade.[3] Smoking is so likely to begin in adolescence that health officials often refer to it as a "pediatric disease."[4] While only adults die from the disease, the disease process begins with the first experimentation with tobacco, usually around age twelve. However, if you can persuade your daughter to avoid smoking until she is twenty-one, it's highly unlikely she will ever take up the habit.[5]

> "If we could affect the smoking habits of just one generation, we could see nicotine addiction go the way of smallpox and polio."
>
> —Dr. David Kessler, former director of the
> Food and Drug Administration

Your daughter needs to know that smoking carries devastating health consequences.[6] For example, women are much more likely to become addicted to nicotine, and quitting is excruciatingly hard. About half of teenagers who start smoking will still be smoking in twenty years.[7] Females find it so hard to quit that most smoke for about four more years than males before finally quitting. Women who start smoking in girlhood appear to have the most difficulty quitting among all types of smokers.[8] Gina is typical of women who sorely regret taking up smoking. She is the mother of a thirteen-year-old daughter, Shannon.

"Shannon doesn't smoke, nor do any of her friends. Unfortunately, I do," admits Gina. "She is beginning to understand the impact it has had on my health; that it is the most addictive substance that is legally available; that my voice has changed tremendously; that my stamina isn't good; that I've tried quitting without success; that I began smoking as a fifteen-year-old who was uneducated about the potential and likely consequences of smoking. I'm a textbook case of a teenager who smoked due to peer pressure and became quickly addicted—although I hadn't a clue at the time."

Gina hopes that Shannon will reject pressures to smoke. And perhaps the knowledge that her mother so regrets starting to smoke will help Shannon reject the practice. Certainly many girls can look at their mothers or grandmothers and see the devastation that smoking has caused. Lung cancer rates among women have increased almost 400 percent in the past thirty years, almost entirely due to more women smoking.[9]

Cigarette smoking is linked to about 90 percent of all lung cancer cases.[10] Smoking increases the rate of other cancers, too, including cancer of the mouth, pancreas, uterus, cervix, kidney, and bladder. Heart disease, stroke, and chronic obstructive lung disease are also caused by smoking. Smoking appears to accelerate bone loss related to osteoporosis and can hasten its onset. Women smokers have nearly twice the death rates from these diseases as do women who have never smoked.[11] Half of all lifelong smokers will die because of the habit.

Judy's family had a long family history of smoking. Her grandmother developed cancer of the larynx and died of the disease. The pain that smoking has caused members of her family has helped Judy and her husband, Mike, focus their efforts on preventing their daughter, Mindi, ten, from ever smoking. "We have always been very open about the dangers of smoking and what can happen if she ever made this choice. My husband and I do

Girls Heavy Use of Cigarettes

As many as one-third of all adolescent girls are smokers.

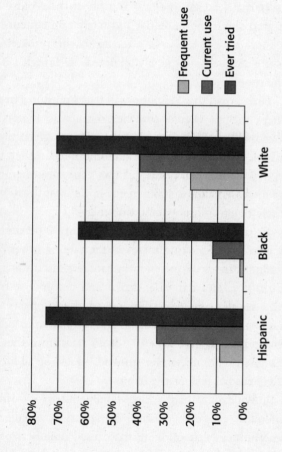

Legend:
- Frequent use
- Current use
- Ever tried

Categories: Hispanic, Black, White

Source: Youth Risk Behavior Surveillance, 1995, MMWR 45(55-5) 1996.

not smoke and I hope, by our example, that we have broken the pattern of smoking in our family."

"When adolescents begin to experiment with cigarettes, they don't understand how difficult it is for smokers to quit. This only becomes evident after they have become addicted smokers."

—Elizabeth Gilpin, professor of Family and
Preventive Medicine, University of California,
San Diego

Make your daughter aware that the consequences of smoking are not just apparent late in life. Young women who smoke may experience significant dilemmas surrounding fertility and pregnancy. For example, a woman who smokes loses the option of using oral contraceptives for birth control since the pill cannot be used safely by smokers. A smoker in her twenties or thirties who wishes to become pregnant has an increased chance of experiencing problems with fertility. And smokers are also twice as likely to have miscarriages. Smokers who do become pregnant must quit or face the real possibility that they could bring harm to their babies. Babies born to smokers are more likely to have lower birth weights and other serious problems. Yet, only about 40 percent of women are able to stop smoking during pregnancy.[12]

Smoking is also linked to a number of other health problems in youth, such as poor nutrition and lack of exercise. This makes sense. A kid who is smoking is less likely to feel good or strong while exercising. Smoking may even be used as a substitute for food.

Smoking even a few cigarettes a day has been shown to stunt the growth of teenagers' lungs so that they hold less air.[13] Girls tend to suffer greater lung deficits from smoking, possibly because they are usually smaller and have narrower airways than boys. Girls also develop wheezing easier than boys who smoke. Smoking also has an immediate effect on teens by increasing the rates of chest illnesses, chronic coughs, and bronchitis.[14] Michelle's daughter, Elizabeth, fourteen, learned quickly that smoking is not innocuous. "A few of Elizabeth's friends smoke, and she did try it. It made her extremely ill. It is our belief, and the belief of our family doctor, that she could be allergic to a chemical in tobacco. She was told about this and told that smoking, especially in her case, could be very dangerous for her health. Her experience with getting so sick was good negative reinforcement for not smoking," says Michelle.

Smoking also seems to trigger permanent genetic changes in teens that increase the risk of lung cancer, even if the teen only smoked for a short time. And, the earlier the smoker starts, the worse the physiological effects. Damage to the lungs is more severe in people who start smoking in their twenties, making the consequences of starting young even more perilous. "It looks like it is the age when smoking starts that is important. It didn't matter if they were heavy or light smokers—what mattered is that they started young," said John Wiencke, a genetics expert at the University of California, San Francisco, who conducted a study demonstrating this effect.

Smoking is linked to other things that are harder to explain. Smokers are less likely to go to college and more likely to divorce. It may be that kids who smoke take on adult roles prematurely but are less likely to succeed in those adult roles.[15] Smoking also dramatically increases the risk that a child will go on to use alcohol or illegal drugs.

Why Girls Start Smoking

Perhaps the major reason that kids experiment with smoking is because they see themselves as immune from any harm. Your daughter may be tempted to try smoking, for example, because she believes she can quit at any time (a serious error in thinking). While it's not clear when nicotine addiction actually begins, it is likely to happen within the first three years of starting to smoke.[16]

Kids begin smoking because it looks appealing.[17] They think smokers are cool or good at sports or thin. Fifth graders who perceive smoking as cool are much more likely to start smoking later on. However, by high school age, most kids have rejected the notion that smoking is attractive. Says Linsey, age sixteen: "I don't think the girls who smoke look any cooler than those who don't."

Kids may choose to smoke because they feel the habit gives them a unique individuality.[18] They also use tobacco for the same reasons some use alcohol or drugs—to satisfy the need to rebel, feel independent, or seek excitement. They appreciate the instant gratification and apparent harmlessness of smoking. This is true of both boys and girls.

A pivotal reason why girls in particular may smoke, however, is because they see cigarettes as diet aids that will help keep them slender.[19] White girls are more likely to embrace this concept compared to other ethnic or racial groups. Tobacco companies have encouraged this fallacious idea and use it in their marketing by naming products with words that include "slim" or "thin," and in ads that show extremely thin models. As many as two-thirds of girls also say they started smoking because of stress. Likewise, girls who are anxious or sad are prone to smoke.[20] Girls with depression are twice as likely to smoke.

Be wary if your daughter has friends who smoke. Kids are especially prone to peer pressure in the early adolescent ages. Terry's fourteen-year-old daughter was caught smoking on school grounds and was disciplined at school and at home. "She was terrified that she was caught smoking. I feel she was influenced by the other kids there. She is very much a follower. She would not have initiated such a plan but would be the first to participate." Another mother, Carole, is also worried that the prevalence of smoking in her community will influence her daughter, Kristen, fifteen. "We don't smoke, and her friends don't smoke. But all their parents do, and this concerns me because I know that kids learn to do what their parents *do,* not what they *say.*"

You will play a big role in whether your daughter decides to smoke. A girl's relationship to her parents in early and middle childhood has a strong impact on her actions and attitudes. Parents who are extremely supportive of their daughters, are warm and encouraging, give positive feedback and physical affection tend to have a good effect on their daughter's decisions regarding smoking.[21] Parents who get along well with their children and know what's going on in their lives and where they are at any given time tend to have fewer substance-using children.[22] You also need to make it clear to your daughter that smoking is unacceptable. David says that he and his wife reinforce a family no-smoking policy even though their daughter Stephanie, eleven, has already expressed her dislike of smoking. "We have taught her that our family doesn't do that. We don't believe that people who smoke are bad, they are just hurting their bodies."

If you smoke, be cognizant that your daughter is more likely to reflect your practices than adhere to your admonitions not to smoke. Even preschoolers whose mothers smoke have been found to be six times more likely to start smoking later in life than those with parents who do not smoke.[23] These preschoolers are likely to conclude that if Mom smokes, then it must be okay or cool.

There is even some evidence, although preliminary, that smoking during pregnancy affects the fetus in such a way that physically predisposes the child to take up smoking more than a decade or two later.[24] If this proves true, efforts to help our daughters avoid smoking can help create a generational chain reaction that could free future generations from addiction.

"Parents don't realize how much they influence their kids. They think they can tell their kids 'I smoke but you shouldn't,' and that will be enough—but it isn't. Those influences are hard to undo."
—Dr. Christine L. Williams, director of the
Child Health Center at the American Health
Foundation

Finally, smoking advertising has a huge impact on youngsters.[25] For example, smoking rates among girls soared around 1967, when cigarette manufacturers began to target advertisements to them, such as with the wildly popular Virginia Slims brand. Tobacco companies are targeting advertising to your children—not you—which means it appears in places where youths congregate, and it is done in a way that catches their eyes. Studies have shown that teens tend to smoke one of three major brands—probably a consequence of heavy advertising by manufacturers of those brands. Bill has tried to help his three teen daughters stop smoking by emphasizing how cigarette manufacturers try to lure people into an unhealthy habit. "I am very honest about smoking and tell them that millions are spent to convince children that smoking is an adult habit when, in fact, smoking is a teen addiction. Almost all smokers started out as children, and I don't know any adult who smokes out of choice."

Prevention

While this grim picture may help you redouble your efforts to prevent your child from smoking, the statistics won't necessarily convince your daughter. But there is so much you can do to make your daughter's decision never to smoke an easier one.

Because kids form their opinions on how smoking looks early, it is imperative to begin talking about smoking prevention no later than third grade. By fifth grade, some perceptions are already formed. Make sure your discussion of smoking doesn't constitute nagging not to do it. Encourage your daughter to think and talk about why people smoke.[26] The discussion should include facts about why smoking is harmful and how tobacco advertisers prey on young people. Tell her that there is no scientific evidence that shows smoking is a useful weight-control device among teens. In fact, smoking to control weight usually backfires because when women do finally quit, they typically gain weight.

Your daughter needs to understand how addictive nicotine is. Within ten seconds of inhaling, nicotine reaches the brain. This rapid, repeated delivery of nicotine to the brain is a major reason why smoking can quickly become addictive.[27] Says Nancy, whose daughter is eleven: "I don't think she'll ever start smoking. We've talked with her about how we started smoking when we were teens, and how very hard it was for us to give it up."

If your daughter seems unimpressed by the threat of developing diseases later in life due to smoking, review all the reasons why smoking hurts her right now. For example, smoking dramatically increases skin wrinkles in women. Point out to your daughter how a friend or acquaintance looks who has smoked for many years. It may be an effective way of getting her to think about the obvious harm from smoking. Remind her that smoking causes bad breath and stained teeth. Girls will take note of these things. Says Maria, age sixteen: "I think smoking is very nasty and unattractive for both boys and girls. I know a lot of guys who wouldn't date girls because they smoke. They wouldn't want to kiss them or be around them and smell like smoke."

You also need to make sure that your daughter feels good enough about herself to resist peer pressure to smoke. Because some kids take up smoking to differentiate themselves from others, you can help prevent smoking by encouraging your daughter to stand out from the crowd in a more positive way—such as through achievement in a sport, art form, or other activity. When you think about it, allowing your daughter to dye her hair orange is a relatively harmless way to acquiesce to her need to feel different or special, compared to her taking up smoking.

Treatment

If your daughter does start smoking, resist the urge to nag her to quit or force her to quit. She will probably just smoke where you can't see it. But set rules, such as forbidding her to smoke in the house or car. After all, her smoking harms the health of others. Continue to express your heartfelt concern for her and keep talking to her about how dangerous smoking is. Keep in mind that research shows that teens have a hard time quitting smoking, although they tend to be more successful at cessation than adults.[28]

Sadly, there is a paucity of research on how to best help teenage smokers quit. But be patient and persistent and look for a cessation program that reports some success with young people.

NOTE: Beware of smoking prevention materials that are produced by cigarette makers or the tobacco industry. While the materials claim to try to deter smoking among youth, leading health authorities have charged that the materials can actually make smoking seem more attractive to kids. For example, one program encourages parents to tell their children not to smoke but to explain that they themselves smoke "because I enjoy smoking." In fact, 75 percent of all adult smokers wish they could quit.

Women tend to start smoking and keep smoking for different reasons than men, so it may be helpful to look for a smoking cessation program that is sensitive to women.

If your daughter has smoked for a year or more, quitting can produce side effects such as severe premenstrual syndrome. Quitting may also cause temporary moodiness and might make her very difficult to live with for a while. But make a sincere effort to help your daughter quit. By eighteen, your daughter will have more independence and autonomy and may begin to resist any pressure to quit. Moreover, some physiological changes that occur after eighteen appear to make quitting even harder.[29] Help your daughter to feel good about her efforts to quit by reminding her about research that shows that, after she quits, her body will bounce back and heal itself from the damaging effects of smoking.

Questions to Ask Your Doctor

- My daughter smokes about once a week, usually when she attends a social event with friends. Could this much smoking lead to an addiction?
- My daughter says she can't and won't stop smoking. I've agreed to stop asking her to quit if she smokes "light" cigarettes. Will these cigarettes help prevent addiction or damage to her health?
- My daughter wants to stop smoking. Can you guide us to an effective cessation program for teenage girls?
- I want to stop smoking in order to set a good example for my daughter. Where can I get information on cessation?
- My daughter won't attend a cessation program but says she will try nicotine gum or the nicotine patch. Are those methods safe for teenagers?
- I smelled heavy cigar smoke on my daughters' clothes last week. She told me that all the kids smoke cigars at parties—just for fun.

She doesn't smoke cigarettes and only smokes a cigar occasionally. Could she still become addicted to nicotine?

Resources

- A wonderful brochure for kids is available through the National Institute on Drug Abuse. It's entitled *Mind Over Matter: The Brain's Response to Nicotine*. Contact 800-729-6686 and ask for publication No. 98-4248.
- A good book for girls that emphasizes effective ways to deal with peer pressure is *My Feelings, My Self*, by Lynda Madaras (Newmarket Press, 1993).
- For more information on smoking prevention or cessation contact the American Cancer Society at 800-ACS-2345 or at www.cancer.org
- Girls and Women Against Tobacco, is a Berkeley, California, organization that is trying to raise awareness of the tobacco industry's attempts to target young women. For a fact sheet or other information call 510-841-6434.
- Girls Inc. offers a program called Friendly PEERsuasion that helps kids learn how they can avoid tobacco and other drugs. Call 212-509-2000, call a Girls Inc. office chapter near your home, or visit www.girlsinc.org.
- The American Lung Association has information on smoking cessation. Call 800-LUNG-USA.
- Information on smoking is available from the Action on Smoking and Health. Visit the web site at www.ash.org or call 202-659-4310.
- Captain Kid Kad Travels to Smokey Island is a web site for kids offering facts about smoking. Visit www.bu.edu/cohis/kids/kidkad/smokey.htm.
- SGR 4 Kids Magazine is a web site for kids encouraging them to make the world smoke free. Visit www.cdc.gov/tobacco/sgr4kids/sgrmenu.htm.

- CDCS Tips for Kids is a web site for kids that tells why the popular band Boyz II Men is smoke free. Visit www.cdc.gov/tobacco/tipskids.htm.
- The American Cancer Society sponsors an annual Great American Smokeout to help people quit. The related web site offers information on smoking, including sound clips from celebrities speaking out against smoking. Visit www.cancer.org/smokeout.

CHAPTER 18

Substance Abuse:
An Equal Opportunity Problem

I N 1999, five Pennsylvania high school girls—best friends—
spent several hours one week at school making a health video
about the dangers of smoking.[1] Ten days later, the girls were
killed when their car slammed into a utility pole. They had
been shopping for prom dresses—and experimenting with a
dangerous drug. Investigators found a can of "Duster II," a
spray used to clean computer keyboards, in the car and, later,
traces of a chemical called difluoroethane in blood samples of
four of the girls. After preaching against the use of one type of
substance, nicotine, the girls succumbed to the temptation to
use another.

"Many girls feel that they don't belong anywhere or with anyone, so they begin to act insensibly and thus run into trouble. Many girls will do anything so they can be cool and belong to a group. For example, some may try drugs so their friends will like them."

—"Gillian," age fifteen, from the American
Association of University Women, Voices of
a New Generation, 1999

Drug use has increased dramatically twice in U.S. history. One surge occurred in the late 1970s. The second major peak has been in the 1990s—specifically, from about 1991 to 1997.[2] But there is a very important difference between these two waves of drug use. In the 1970s, neither parents nor educators nor health officials knew much about what to do to prevent the devastating trend. Today, after twenty years of research, we know a lot more about why kids use drugs and what we can do to prevent it.[3] Adults today have a much poorer excuse for allowing drug abuse to occur. We have strategies to prevent it. And we can prevent it in our cherished daughters. The most recent surveys even show a small drop in the numbers of kids using drugs, suggesting that efforts to prevent substance abuse do work.

The Facts

While drug use appears to be declining slightly in the late 1990s, too many kids still use drugs. Drug use occurs among all, kinds of kids, from all ethnic groups and all income levels. African-American and Latino youths tend to be initiating drug use at higher rates than Caucasian youths.[4]

Girls, more so than boys, are likely to use "socially appropriate" drugs, like alcohol and marijuana, when they are with other girls. Many won't use illicit drugs, like stimulants or cocaine,

The Monitoring the Future Study is a project by the University of Michigan to track youth drug use patterns on an annual basis. This chart shows a steady increase in drug use from 1991 to 1997. In 1998, however, there were slight drops in the numbers of children using drugs.

Students using any illicit drug	1991	1995	1997	1998
8th graders	18.7%	28.5%	29.4%	29.0%
10th graders	30.6%	40.9%	47.3%	44.9%
12th graders	44.1%	48.4%	54.3%	54.1%

Source: University of Michigan, Monitoring the Future Study, 1999.

unless introduced to the substance by boys, usually within the context of a dating relationship.[5] While many parents fear that their children will experiment with deadly substances like cocaine or heroin, it is much more important for you to do your best to prevent your daughter from experimenting with tobacco, alcohol, and marijuana. These are the substances she is most likely to be offered, and using any of these drugs increases the risk that she will try other drugs. The typical pattern among kids who use drugs is that they start by using tobacco and alcohol then move to marijuana and other drugs. Smoking and drinking are not the cause of later drug use, and not all kids who smoke or drink use other substances. Nevertheless, the link between smoking and drinking and later drug use is striking. Children who smoke or drink are sixty-five times more likely to move on to other drugs than those who never smoke or drink. Thus, it is imperative to make sure your prevention efforts are focused foremost on the avoidance of smoking and alcohol early in life.[6]

Alcohol

Alcohol presents a particular challenge for many families because alcohol is a legal drug and many adults consume it. If you or your spouse drink, it is very important to make sure your daughter witnesses only responsible drinking, including limiting intake and never drinking and driving. Even with this practice, you may have a hard time convincing a teenager that it's okay for you to drink but not for her. Your daughter, at ages eight through twelve, may scold you about drinking. But she may be tempted, eventually, to mimic your practices. "Annie is funny about alcohol. If she sees me having a glass of wine or my husband having a beer she gets a little upset. We explain to her that alcohol in moderation and used by responsible adults is all right. But that children who are still growing and aren't able to responsibly drink aren't to drink," says Tammy, whose daughter is eight. If your daughter questions your drinking, you could point out that alcohol is legal and can be consumed safely by adults without causing disease although you realize that drinking alcohol is not a healthy habit. In addition, explain that underage drinking is a crime.

Families with a history of alcoholism need to be particularly cognizant about the risks of drinking. Eve, the mother of Susanna, age nine, has explained the family's history when admonishing her daughter that drinking will pose special risks to her. "There is a history of alcoholism on both sides of my family. I will tell her everything except the most disgusting details, with the hope that she will comprehend the insidious nature of alcoholism."

The vast majority of high school seniors have tried alcohol, and many have their first drink around age fourteen.[7] The pressure to drink begins even earlier. About 26 percent of fourth graders and 40 percent of sixth graders say they know of peers who have tried beer or wine.[8] While teen boys used to drink alcohol more than girls, girls have caught up over the past decade.[9] In the years from 1993 to 1998, drinking among tenth-grade girls increased 38 percent. If this trend continues, girls will soon be heavier drinkers than boys. The increasing rates of alcohol use among girls don't bode well for the future health of women. Early use of alcohol is a very strong predictor of the development of a serious alcohol problem later in life.[10]

Another worrisome trend is girls' tendency to drink large quantities at one time. Bingeing is defined as having five or more drinks on one occasion. In 1997, one in four twelfth-grade girls admitted to binge drinking.[11] A major study by the American Academy of Pediatrics found that 16 percent of teens who drink experience "black-outs," where they cannot remember what happened while drinking. Surveys taken on college campuses show that bingeing is a huge problem and leads to higher rates of rape, assault, and sexually transmitted diseases. In the past fifteen years, the number of college women who say they drink with the intention of getting drunk has tripled.[12]

Why do kids drink? Part of the reason has to do with the availability of alcohol in our culture and its acceptance by adults, many of whom also drink. Kids also say they drink to relax, have fun, and fit in with friends.[13] Smaller numbers of kids say they drink to try to feel happy or forget their problems or even to get drunk. Among girls, the major reasons for using alcohol are to fit in with other kids and because of peer pressure. This fact weighs on the mind of Judy, whose daughter is twelve: "I am concerned because even the strongest, smartest kid can fall prey to others' proddings."

Heavy Alcohol Use Reported by More Girls

Many high school girls try alcohol and a growing number report episodic heavy drinking (five or more drinks at one time).

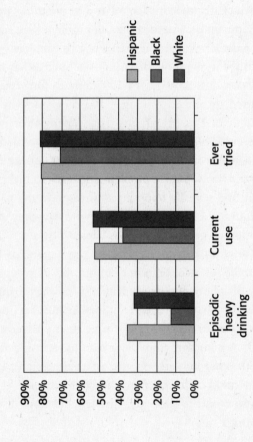

Hispanic
Black
White

Source: Youth Risk Behavior Surveillance, MMWR 45(55-4), 1996.

A Special Note about Drunk Driving

"My whole family drinks. I have a drink or two at times. But I never drink a whole bottle."

—Patrice, age fifteen

Many teens use or experiment with alcohol. You should persist in your efforts to forbid your daughter to use alcohol before she is twenty-one and can make her own decision. However, it is also important to make it clear to your daughter that the mistake of using alcohol is greatly compounded by the decision to drive while drinking or ride in a car with a driver who has been drinking. Nearly half of all traffic accidents nationwide are alcohol-related, with about 18 percent of those drivers ages sixteen to twenty. About 2.5 million teens drive while under the influence of alcohol.[14]

It may seem to be a contradiction, but it's okay to tell your daughter, "Don't ever drink. But if you do drink and cannot safely get home, call me and I will come and get you." Then promise not to scream or punish your daughter when you pick her up. But make it clear that you and your daughter will sit down the following day for a discussion on why she is using alcohol and why you object. The goal of this is, first and foremost, to protect her from a serious car accident. You can then tackle the issue of persuading her to avoid drugs.

This is a must-rule in every household. Every day, about eight teens die in alcohol-related car accidents. You can try other approaches as well. Draw up a written contract (have your daughter write it) that spells out your family policy on drinking and driving. Ask your daughter to sign and honor the contract. In the contract, parents should also promise that when called to pick up your daughter, you will come, no questions asked. Post the contract on a refrigerator or in some prominent place at home. Have regular family discussions about drunk driving. Sadly, there is news every few months about kids in your community killed from driving drunk. Discuss the cases with your daughter. Have her read the newspaper articles.

A recent survey found that two-thirds of teens establish a designated driver when out drinking with friends.[15] The problem is that they tend to think that as long as they have a designated driver, drinking is okay. A tragic car accident in Newport Beach, California, suggests this belief is a fallacy. In that incident, a van loaded with drinking teens, but driven by a teen who agreed to be the designated driver and remained sober, careened out of control down a curving road, killing two and seriously injuring several others. Although the driver was sober, the exuberant carelessness and wild behavior apparently affected everyone in the car—sober or not.

Marijuana

Marijuana is the most commonly used illegal drug. Use of this drug has soared among high school youths since 1991.[16] Half of all kids try marijuana before graduating from high school, and its use is increasing faster among girls than boys.[17] The average age of first using marijuana is fourteen. Kids typically try marijuana because they are curious or because so many kids are using it that they feel compelled to try and fit in. Kids who use marijuana may seem dizzy or have trouble walking. They act silly, have red or bloodshot eyes, or have a hard time remembering things.

> "When I would sit down and try to figure something out it was like my brain would stop working."
>
> —Teen girl from the videotape *Marijuana: What Can Parents Do?*, U.S. Department of Health and Human Services

Inhalants

Inhalant use, like that which killed the five Pennsylvania girls, is also increasingly common and deadly. Called "huffing" among kids, it ranks fourth among all forms of drug use by teens (about 17 percent of teens say they have tried it), and is especially popular among seventh and eighth graders. And, like other drugs, girls are increasing their use of inhalants faster than boys.[18] Inhalant use is tempting for younger kids and for those who might not otherwise use drugs because the chemicals are legal and easy to find. Spray-can solvents, typewriter correction fluid, spray paint, air freshener, vegetable cooking spray, and other products are used by kids to get a quick high from inhaling the fumes. More than 1,000 products contain euphoriant inhalants. Huffing can cause sudden cardiac arrest.

Other Illicit Drugs

Hallucinogens are substances like LSD, MDMA (also called ecstasy), or PCP (also called angel dust). LSD is the most common hallucinogen. It can cause sleeplessness, raised heart rate and blood pressure, and severe emotional reactions, such as terror. As many as 12 percent of high school seniors say they have tried LSD.[19]

Steroids are drugs derived from hormones. While steroids can be useful medicines for people with certain health problems, they have been misused increasingly over the last decade by athletes who think that steroids will help their athletic performance. While boys are more prone to try steroids, an increasing number of female athletes also admit they use steroids. There are many dangers to steroid use. In women, steroids can cause masculinization, such as the growth of facial hair and deepening of the voice, menstrual cycle changes, breast reduction, acne, and other problems. Steroids change cholesterol and blood pressure levels, damage joints, and increase the risk of injury and cancer. Use in adolescents can halt growth. Steroids also cause changes in behavior and emotions, including increasing anxiety, jealousy, and anger.

Methamphetamine is a powerful addictive stimulant that typically causes deep despair and regret in people who use it. It is made in clandestine laboratories and is popular in particular regions of the country. Called ice or meth or speed, it causes severe addiction and can lead to violent behavior, anxiety, and insomnia. Chronic use can damage the heart and lead to death by overdose. Methamphetamine is commonly distributed at so-called rave parties.

Drug use has such severe consequences that it's no wonder parents worry so much about it. Kids who use drugs are prone to all types of serious accidents, including car accidents. They make poor decisions about sex and increase their risk of pregnancy, sexually transmitted diseases, and rape. Drug use increases the risk of homicide, suicide, and nonfatal forms of violence. It leads to delinquency and crime. In a less tangible way, drug use undermines the very development of a girl. It can impair the growth of her identity and limit her ability to handle the tasks and demands of adolescence. If she stumbles in this process, the deficits in her development can affect her later success in relationships, marriage, parenting, and career advancement. Substance abuse also interferes with a girl's ability to identify and cope with her feelings. For example, instead of being able to recognize that she feels nervous or depressed, she may instead gloss over her feelings and tell herself only that she needs a beer or a joint.

Why Kids Use Drugs

The path to drug abuse begins very early for some children. There are major home influences that can begin to affect even a very young child and predispose her to substance abuse. If you recognize any of these three situations in your family, it's important to seek professional guidance so that you can help prevent the development of psychological and behavioral problems in your daughter, like drug use.

The major risk factors that occur *early* in a child's life include:

- Chaotic home environments, particularly in which parents abuse substances or suffer from mental illnesses
- Ineffective parenting (such as being highly authoritarian or ignoring objectional behavior), especially with children with difficult temperaments and conduct disorders
- Lack of mutual attachments and nurturing

In girls especially, problems at home or a poor relationship with parents tends to raise the risk of drug use. Drug use also tends to go hand in hand with other problems, such as sexual abuse, domestic violence among parents, and mental illness. It has only been very recently that health experts have begun to understand that many kids who use drugs may themselves be mentally ill and are attempting to "self-medicate" through their drug use. Children who have conduct or oppositional disorders, eating disorders, depression, and anxiety disorders are much more likely to use drugs. Conduct disorder, which is behavior that repeatedly violates rules and the rights of others, is a particularly devastating disorder that dramatically raises the risk of drug use. Conduct disorder is less common in girls than in boys. Any evaluation of why a girl is using drugs should include an exploration of whether she may be depressed, anxious, have attention deficit disorder, or some other mental or behavioral problem.

The second grouping of risk factors appears a little later in a girl's life, when she is beginning to socialize outside the family. These risk factors have less to do with a girl's family life. In other words, even if you have a stable, happy, and loving home, your daughter could be influenced by one or more of these other risk factors that lead to experimentation with drugs. These include:[20]

- Inappropriately shy or aggressive behavior in the classroom
- Failure in school performance
- Poor social coping skills
- Affiliations with peers who consistently misbehave
- Perceptions of approval of drug-using behaviors in the school, peer, and community environments

Kids also use drugs for other obvious reasons, such as if drug use is prevalent in the community (either using or trafficking) or if their friends use drugs. Certainly, hanging around with antisocial kids who have problems in school and with authorities is a red flag for possible drug use. "I am concerned about alcohol for my sixteen-year-old," says Katie, who also has an eleven-year-old girl. "The clique at her high school drinks, and I don't like for her to hang around with the 'in' crowd. So the message we give our girls is don't do it, and we will find out if you do it!"

Drug use often begins when children are experiencing vulnerable transitions in their lives. One of the most common transitions is the movement from elementary to middle school or junior high. In middle school, children are likely to encounter drugs for the first time and may also often feel very self-conscious about the need to socialize and fit it. A second vulnerable period is in high school. Teens may start using drugs because of worries about the future or current problems and pressures. They view drugs as a way to escape from their worries. Girls are much more likely than boys to turn to substances as a way of soothing stress and avoiding their problems.

The media also reinforces the idea that drug use is acceptable and that our culture is a substance-using one. Teens who watch a lot of TV and music videos are more likely to start drinking, perhaps due to the steady exposure of drinking portrayals (which are usually positive).[21] A study of fifty animated movies, for example, showed that tobacco or alcohol was used by at least one character in 68 percent of the movies.[22] Moreover, the Internet has afforded new opportunities for alcohol and tobacco companies to market to vulnerable groups, such as children and teens. One survey of twenty-eight web sites on beer products found that 82 percent had features that would appeal to youth, such as cartoon-like characters, games, contests, and free prizes of merchandise that kids covet.[23] While many of the sites state that participants should be twenty-one or older, that admonition may make it even more appealing to some kids.

Acceptance of alcohol is everywhere in our culture. Even the retailer Abercrombie & Fitch, which markets to teen and college youth, inserted a theme in a 1998 catalog called "Drinking 101." It portrayed alcohol use as a major part of campus life.[24] Angry protests from parents, educators, and health professionals led the company to pull the ads and issue an apology.

To help counteract the messages that your daughter gets from media sources, teach her to objectively assess what she hears or sees. For example, if a commercial comes on showing young women having a good time drinking, you might comment that the commercial is by a wine company that is trying to convince people to buy its product. Point out that the ad doesn't show how the women will get home or if they have a designated driver or whether some of the women have chosen to have a soft drink rather than the wine.[25]

Stress Impacts Girls Health

Girls say stress is a major reason why they use drugs, smoke or drink. This chart shows the percentage of girls giving reasons for their behavior.

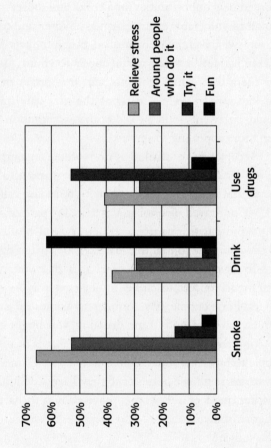

Source: Commonwealth Fund.

Preventing Drug Use

Lawrence and Allison have already begun to talk to Devon, age ten, about the pervasive use of drugs among kids. "We have discussed that parties will not be attended unless I know of adequate supervision and that my husband and I will also drop in sporadically to see what is happening. Drugs under no circumstances will be tolerated in our home as long as we are responsible for her," says Allison. Establishing a hard line early in your daughter's life is a good way to start. It's a lot easier to prevent drug use than to try to deal with it after risk factors have already appeared. When your daughter is young, begin thinking about these factors that have proven to reduce the chance that she will use drugs:[26]

- Strong bonds with the family
- Experience of parental monitoring with clear rules of conduct within the family unit and involvement of parents in the lives of their children
- Success in school performance
- Strong bonds with prosocial institutions, such as the family, school, and religious organizations
- Adoption of conventional norms about drug use

You should have many discussions with your daughter about drug use, from the time she is five or six to the late teen years. It may sometimes seem as if you are a broken record and that she is bored with hearing it. But, in fact, repeating an anti-drug abuse message has been shown to work. The more parents talk about it, the less likely kids are to use drugs.[27] Kids who hear nothing from their parents about the topic, however, are much more likely to use drugs.

One of the most effective things you can tell your daughter is that not everyone does drugs and that doing drugs is not the social norm.[28] It's also very clear that girls who are involved in challenging, fun, and stimulating activities (such as music instruction, sports, or various clubs) are less likely to be using drugs. Mary says she intends to keep Natasha, thirteen, very busy. "I am hoping that by keeping her very involved in after-school activities she will not have time for drugs." And, in the home of Walt and Vicki, sports is emphasized to remind Billie, age thirteen, that her body is to be cherished, not abused. "I'm hoping she will be very much into the fitness thing and won't be interested in polluting her body," says Vicki.

Let your daughter blame you for the strict limits she is under, such as by saying "Go ahead and tell your friends that I said you had to be home by eleven P.M." Ashley, thirteen, puts it this way: "My mom and dad talked to me about this stuff. I don't think I will do alcohol or drugs or smoke or anything like that because if they found out they would probably kill me."

Talk to your daughter about the drug scene at her school. Ask her who uses drugs, where kids get drugs, and whether there is pressure to try drugs. This creates a forum for your daughter to ask questions of her own, express her concerns, or clarify the family's rules and beliefs. Make sure you don't turn discussions into lectures. More than half of the discussion should consist of you listening to what your daughter has to say.

Kids have opportunities to experiment with drugs— a fact that parents find hard to face.

Teens who said they tried marijuana: 42%
Parents who think it's possible that their kids have tried marijuana: 14%

Teens who said they had been offered marijuana: 53%
Parents who consider it likely that their teens will be offered marijuana: 37%

Source: Partnership for a Drug-Free America.

"Kids who are learning nothing at home about drugs are using drugs at far higher rates. We're asking parents to consider that they don't know their teenagers as well as they think they do."

—Steve Dnistrian, Partnership for a Drug-Free America

How much should schools do to prevent drug use? That question is heavily debated. Some research suggests that popular programs like D.A.R.E. don't have a long-term impact on children's decisions to use drugs. Other experts strongly believe in the program and others similar to it. What seems to be most important is that children receive drug-use prevention education at both home and school. Part of the prevention effort should include teaching kids about the negative effects of drugs. This is something that school programs can do very well. But that effort will be meaningless if children do not hear prevention messages at home and have good role models in their parents. Take advantage of your school's drug education weeks by reinforcing the message at home and by asking your daughter, every day, what she has learned and discussed. Use this as an opportunity to make your family's values and rules clear.

What to Do If Your Daughter Is Using Drugs

Martha, whose daughters are sixteen and seventeen, hopes her girls will steer clear of drugs. But that doesn't mean she will shut her eyes to symptoms of possible use. "I don't believe either girl has tried any illegal substances or alcohol or would do so. That said, I know it's pretty common to be fooled by your kids. It is a concern."

It's important to detect drug use early, before your daughter is placed in danger. But how do you do that? Studies show that it is particularly hard for girls and women to acknowledge that they have a substance abuse problem and to seek help. Many either deny they need treatment or are ashamed of their problem.[29] In 1999, the federal government released guidelines designed to help parents, doctors, teachers, and other authority figures recognize the signs of possible drug use and intervene. These warning signs include major behavior changes, psychological difficulties, emergency room hospital visits for injuries or gastrointestinal disturbances, sudden changes in grades, unexplained school absences, and the tendency to be accident prone. If you are not sure how to evaluate your daughter for signs of drug use, enlist the help of a physician who is familiar with these guidelines.

You're not alone if you're dealing with a child using drugs. About 77,000 teens under age eighteen are in substance abuse treatment each year (a figure that has doubled since 1991).[30] Unfortunately, most kids enter treatment for drug abuse only after they have suffered some serious consequence, such as getting arrested or having a car accident or overdosing.

How do you approach your child? According to the new guidelines, parents should avoid a punitive, heavy-handed approach. Being angry or bossy tends to backfire by straining relationships between parents and kids. Instead, try a loving, subtle, "motivational" approach. Try to reach out to your daughter with reassurances of your love, support, and concern. Don't yell, accuse, make threats, or label your daughter as an addict or user. If you're not sure if she is using, respectfully ask her. Don't keep your worries to yourself. If you know she is using, talk openly and repeatedly about how worried you are and how much you want to help your daughter. Don't become angry if your child tries to turn the table by criticizing you for your own use of alcohol or cigarettes. Gently steer the conversation back to her problem. Point out how drug use can hurt her, such as by interfering with her studies, job, or sports participation.[31] Pam found out her daughter had also tried drinking when the family sat down to discuss an incident in which she had been caught with cigarettes. Pam and her husband discussed the family rule that substances were forbidden and told their daughter that she would have to earn back the trust that had been lost. "I believe she stopped drinking," says Pam. "We are building trust again. But this is always a worry and concern."

If you have confirmed that your child is using drugs, schedule an appointment with a mental health professional. You can start by visiting your primary care doctor or pediatrician. If that person is unable to help, contact a child psychologist or child psychiatrist for an evaluation.

The best treatment for your child will probably not be the popular treatment programs for adults, such as 12-step programs. Adult treatment programs tend not to work as well with children. If your daughter needs a residential treatment program, look for one that is less confrontational and more supportive than the programs typically designed for adults. Teens may need longer treatment than adults.

Questions to Ask Your Doctor

- In our culture, it is common to have wine at dinner. Is this setting a bad example for our daughter? Also, we have allowed the teenagers to drink a small glass of wine at dinner. Is this harmful?
- My daughter takes a prescription medication for a particular health problem. What can you tell my daughter and me about the interaction of drugs or alcohol with her medication? Is she in even more danger than other teens who experiment with drugs?
- My daughter has come home intoxicated five times within the last three months. Does this constitute a drinking problem that requires professional treatment?
- My daughter has arrived home from a party and acted odd—tired, stumbling, and uncommunicative. However, I could not detect any

alcohol or marijuana on her breath or clothes. What are the symptoms of other drug use?

- I believe my daughter is smoking marijuana, but she denies it. What can I do to get her to confide in me?
- I found marijuana in my daughter's dresser. How should I confront her?
- Will you talk to my daughter about the dangers of drug use?
- There is a strong history of alcoholism on my side of the family. Does this history place my daughter at higher risk for developing the disease?

Resources

- For information on prevention of alcohol abuse call 800-729-6686 or visit the web site for the National Clearinghouse for Alcohol and Drug Information at www.nida.nih.gov.
- For a copy of the new guidelines on helping children who use drugs, call the National Clearinghouse for Alcohol and Drug Information at 800-487-4889.
- For information on treatment of drug abuse disorders call the Center for Substance Abuse Treatment, an arm of the U.S. Department of Health and Human Services, at 800-662-HELP.
- The National Inhalant Prevention Coalition offers information about inhalants and how to prevent abuse. Visit the web site at www.inhalants.org.
- A helpful book for teens who fear that a friend may have an alcohol or drug problem is available from the Hazelden Center for Youth and Families. Call 800-I-DO-CARE or write the Hazelden Foundation at CO 3 P.O. Box 11, Center City, MN 55012-0011.
- For a pamphlet entitled *Ten Actions Families Can Take to Raise Drug-Free Kids*, visit the web site of the Office of National Drug Control Policy at www.whitehousedrugpolicy.gov.

- Kids who work for a social cause, such as stopping drunk driving, are more likely to abide by their beliefs. Encourage your daughter to join Students Against Drunk Driving. Contact P.O. Box 800, Marlboro, MA 01752, or call 508-481-3568.
- *Under Whose Influence? The Decision Is Yours* is a wonderful book to help preteens deal with social pressures to drink. It's by Judy Link, Parenting Press, Inc., Seattle, WA. Call 800-992-6657.
- *Saying NO Is Not Enough*, by Robert Schwebel (Newmarket Press, 1998), is a helpful guide for parents of children ages three through nineteen in preventing drug use, including smoking and alcohol.
- The National Clearinghouse for Alcohol and Drug Information's For Kids Only web site instructs kids about drugs and how they affect the brain. There is also advice (in English and Spanish) on what to do in different situations to resist drugs. Visit www.health.org/kidsarea/.
- Mind Over Matter is a web site for kids that helps them understand the effects of drugs on the brain. Visit www.nida.nih.gov/MOM/MOMIndex.html.
- Project Know is a site for kids that tests their knowledge about drugs and provides comments from kids who choose not to use drugs. Visit www.projectknow.com/.
- Get It Straight: The Facts About Drugs informs kids about the physical, emotional, financial, and legal consequences of using drugs. Visit www.usdoj.gov/dea/pubs/straight/cover.htm.
- NCADI: A Guide for Teens is a web site to help teens learn what they can do if a friend has a drug problem. Visit www.health.org.

CHAPTER 19

A Safe Environment:
Rules and Responsibility

Ben, Terry, and their daughter, Candie, ten, live in a charming, older section of their large, urban city. While they love some aspects of their home and neighborhood, such as their short commutes to work and school, Ben and Terry have become very worried about the effect of this urban environment on Candie's health. From the exhaust from city buses that run by their house to the lead and asbestos problems at their inner-city school, the family often feels besieged by potential health threats. "My biggest fear for Candie is the environment," says Terry. "We are destroying our environment at a fast and furious pace. And I don't feel we are even aware of all the dangers that face us."

Ben and Terry are right to be concerned. And their knowledge can help them take actions to curtail the environmental threats they face. Indeed, if we are to succeed in our goal to help our daughters avoid many health problems in adulthood, then we must confront the fact that our environment today is far more hazardous than ever before. Accident rates among children and teens remain unacceptably high, and exposures to environmental toxins have dramatically increased among children.

There are so many potential hazards from living in a fast-paced, highly industrialized world that it's natural to feel helpless. Laurie, who has two daughters, admits that she simply hopes for the best when it comes to protecting her girls from environmental hazards. "I don't do much about it. Nowadays, everything is so bad for everyone's health." But you can have a significant impact on protecting your daughter—and future generations of girls—from environmental health threats by adopting three strategies:

1. Establish a set of safety rules in your house and teach your daughter what they are and why you have them.
2. Exercise your consumer shopping skills to purchase products that protect the environment.
3. Become an active citizen with a voice on important environmental issues and legislation.

Maureen, the mother of two teenage girls, says that she has urged her daughters to be responsible for any actions they take that may further degrade the environment. "They know how important it is for everyone to be concerned about our environment. We view it as a valuable gift God has given us that we need to take care of."

Pollution and Chemical Exposures

We live in a world heavily reliant on chemicals. In the past few decades, thousands of new chemicals have been invented and dispersed into our environment through new consumer commodities. Science has shown that high doses of many chemicals impact our health. But almost all of the research has been performed examining adults' exposures to environmental toxins. Far less is known about children's exposures to pollution and chemicals. Even though children are much more vulnerable to the effects of toxic exposures, they have been the least-studied group.

Toxic exposures to children differ from exposures to adults and deserve separate studies and standards, both of which are only recently being undertaken in the United States. The major difference in children is that they are growing and developing.[1] Thus their organs and systems are functioning at different rates than are adults'. Children are also different from adults in the amount and kind of toxic exposures they receive. Children eat more food, drink more water, and breathe more air per pound of body weight than do adults. All this could dramatically increase children's exposure to toxins. Moreover, children's activities place them in closer proximity to chemicals. For example, they spend more time outdoors, getting dirty and running. They place their hands to their mouths more, increasing the possibility that they are introducing toxins into their systems.[2] Since children may be more vulnerable to the effects of toxins than adults receiving a comparable dose, laws that regulate the amount of toxic exposures permissible *should* be based on the health and safety of children. There is a wave of national legislation focusing on this concept that parents should support.

FACT: Asthma is increasing among Americans, especially children, with a whopping 72 percent increase in children from 1982 to 1994.
—National Institute of Allergy and Infectious Diseases.

Air Pollution

In 1995, more than one-quarter of all U.S. children lived in areas that failed to meet federal air quality standards.[3] Air pollution is typically comprised of four harmful substances: ozone, nitrogen dioxide, microscopic particles called particulate matter, and acid vapors. Air pollution increases asthma attacks in children prone to the disorder and damages healthy lungs in all children.

Poor air quality is an enormous threat to our children—particularly our daughters. Boys and girls are both harmed by air pollution, but girls tend to experience a more extreme deficit in lung function.[4] Long-term exposure to airborne toxins can limit the growth of your daughter's lungs.[5] Air pollution is not only caused by such things as cars and smokestacks. Parents who smoke in the home are exposing their daughter to massive amounts of harmful chemicals. "I know that secondhand smoke is bad," admits Patty, the mother of one girl. "I smoke outside, or in the furnace room where there is an air-filtering system next to me."

Landfills

Toxic landfills and hazardous waste sites also pose a threat to our girls. In 1999, the largest school district in the country, Los Angeles Unified, struggled with the decision of whether to build schools on two parcels of property it owned—both hazardous waste sites. As many as four million children live within a mile of a federally designated Superfund hazardous waste disposal site and are at risk of exposure from chemicals leaked into the air, groundwater,

What Parents Can Do about Air Pollution

- Emphasize public transportation and carpooling to reduce air pollution.
- Pay attention to news reports about air quality and limit your daughter's outdoor playtime when levels are high. Close your windows when levels are high.
- Make sure your school has a policy limiting outdoor playtime when air quality is poor.
- Reduce allergens and irritants in your home by cleaning frequently, using and frequently cleaning air filters, and removing drapes and carpets where possible.
- Don't smoke or allow smoking inside your home.

Source: Mothers & Others For a Livable Planet, The Green Guide, July 1, 1998.

and soil.[6] If you know or suspect that you live close to a toxic dump site, you are entitled to information about possible risks to your family's health. Call the regional office of the Environmental Protection Agency for more information. You can also do your part to address the issue of overuse of landfills by recycling waste products.

Lead

Exposure to lead is linked to many devastating problems for children, including impaired attention, hyperactivity, learning disabilities, behavior problems, and decreased IQ scores. Children are harmed by lead levels that are much lower than was thought a decade or two ago. No child should have a blood lead level exceeding 10 ug/dl.[7] But as many as 4 percent of all preschoolers have lead levels over this limit.[8] Lead poisoning doesn't cause overt symptoms, so many parents may be unaware their children are being affected by a preventable and treatable problem.

In the late 1970s lead in the environment was reduced when leaded gasoline was phased out. A major source of lead that remains problematic, however, is lead in paints that were used before 1980. Children who consume chips of flaking, lead-based paint can accumulate dangerous levels of lead in their blood. The vast majority of homes built before 1980 still contain lead paint. Lead can also contaminate drinking water when released from lead solder in pipe joints and lead pipes.

What Parents Can Do about Lead:

- Ask your pediatrician to give your daughter a blood test if you have any fears that she may be exposed to lead.
- Get your home tested for lead if it was built before 1980. You can also purchase kits like Lead Check Swabs (800-262-LEAD) from hardware stores.
- To learn more about how to protect children from lead call the National Safety Council's National Lead Information Center at 800-LEAD-FYI.
- Avoid storing or drinking liquids in lead crystal and serving foods in lead-glazed ceramics.
- Serve your children a diet rich in calcium and iron and low in fat to decrease the absorption of lead.
- Use only very cold tap water for drinking and cooking if you suspect that lead pipes or lead solder may have been used in constructing your home. Hot water is more likely to leach lead out of the pipes.
- Avoid vinyl products, such as backpacks, that may contain lead.

Source: Mothers & Others For a Livable Planet, The Green Guide, July 1, 1998.

Pesticides

We know we should feed our children several servings of fruits and vegetables each day to protect against disease. It is disappointing, however, that we have to worry that the food sources richest in nutrients can be tainted with chemicals that harm health. Pesticides remain a big problem in our nation's supply of produce because of their widespread use in farming and as home insecticides. Children are exposed to pesticides in food, water, from lawn products, or if their parents work around such chemicals. If consumed in high enough quantities, organophosphate pesticides can cause mood changes, insomnia, headaches, nausea, and confusion in children.

You can reduce your child's exposure by carefully washing all fruits and vegetables before eating or cooking or by purchasing organic produce. Avoid using chemicals on your lawn, even if it means your lawn is not quite as green as you would like. Aaron and Pamela have two daughters and one son. They decided when their first child was born that they would no longer use lawn chemicals. "We have well water so we do not use chemical lawn applications. But many of our neighbors still do!" If you do use lawn chemicals, do not allow children to step on the grass until it has been thoroughly washed off. If you do use pesticides, use only EPA-approved chemicals and follow the directions closely.

Since your daughter spends so much of her time in school, you need to care about her school environment as well. Call your children's school or school district office to make sure that organophosphates are not used at the school for pest control.

Water Pollution

Drinking water can contain lead, pesticides, bacteria, and other chemicals. Children drink twice the amount of water as adults and thus are more vulnerable to the effects of consuming unclean water.[9] Drinking water violations are far too common. Most cities have an average of 1.8 violations per year of the Safe Drinking Water Act.[10] Contact your local water utility to receive recent test results and notices of violations. If your city has a problem with water purity, consider installing a good water purification system at home. Another option is to use bottled water, but do some research first to make sure you are actually purchasing water that has been purified. Some bottled water is just tap water. Use cold water when cooking and let water run a minute or so before filling a glass or pan for cooking.

Accidents

Another consequence of living in a high-tech environment is that the possibilities for serious accident have become greater than ever. Unintentional injuries are the leading cause of death in children age fourteen and under.[11] About 8,000 kids a year are killed and 50,000 permanently disabled due to preventable injuries.[12] The major causes of these injuries are motor vehicle accidents (including bicycle and pedestrian mishaps), burns, and drownings. While most injuries and deaths occur to youngsters under age four, older children are not immune from risk. Many accidents among older children occur outdoors.

Look for opportunities to teach safety as your daughter moves through important developmental milestones. For example, when your daughter receives her first bicycle, lay down street safety rules about the use of helmets, where to ride, how to obey traffic regulations, what clothing to wear, and how to look and listen for traffic. Likewise, children who skateboard should wear protective clothing and helmets and have strict rules about where they can board. Children should be limited to the kind of "tricks" they want to try (like jumping ramps) and should be told never to "hitch" the skateboard to the back of a car or bicycle.

Dog bites are a major source of injuries to kids. Teach your child how to deal with pets (both your own pets and pets they may encounter outside the home). There are several books and videos to help kids learn important pet safety rules (see Resources).

The good news is that as many as 90 percent of all unintentional injuries can be prevented.[13] Your daughter should understand that the world can be dangerous *if* we act recklessly or thoughtlessly. Remember that children around age six and younger do not have the ability to think about risks and need much more direct protection. Children at age seven still do not even have the skills that allow good judgment in crossing streets.[14]

> "If a disease were killing our children at the rate unintentional injuries are, the public would be outraged and demand that this killer be stopped."
>
> —Dr. C. Everett Koop, former U.S. Surgeon General, former chairman of the National SAFE Kids Campaign

One of the first things you can do with your young daughter is to teach her how to dial 911 or your area's emergency number. Proceed to everyday matters, such as using seat belts and wearing helmets. Be vigilant all the time while bearing in mind that the majority of accidental deaths occur in warm weather and in the evening when children are out of school and least likely to be supervised.[15] Most injuries also occur in or near the home.

Teaching Girls How to Handle Emergencies

Fire Safety Plan

- Your daughter should know what to do if there is a fire in the house. Show her two ways out of the house.

- Let your daughter hear what the smoke detector sounds like so she won't be frightened by it.
- Explain that crawling is best when the air is smoky.
- Tell her not to try to take a favorite toy or pet from the house during an emergency evacuation.
- Tell your child that she should not hide during a fire. She needs to be aggressive in fleeing from the structure.
- Practice the "stop, drop, and roll" technique to smother flames on clothing.
- Have smoke detectors and check batteries yearly.

Water Safety Plan

- Supervise your child around water and tell her she should leave a pool that is not supervised by an adult.
- Enroll your daughter in swimming lessons when she is a toddler and continue with the lessons until she is a strong swimmer (typically at least five years if you don't have a pool at home).
- Make sure your daughter knows to wear a life vest when participating in boating or water sports.
- Learn CPR and enroll your teen daughter in a CPR class.

Poison Safety Plan

- Tell your child not to eat or drink anything that she finds.
- Show your daughter a prescription medicine bottle and stress that if she ever finds that type of container to bring it to you immediately and never to eat what is in it.
- Be on guard when your daughter is visiting friends' or relatives' homes who do not have children and may not have child-proofed.
- Keep any medicines and toxic chemicals out of young children's reach.
- Keep the local poison control center number near the phone and tell your daughter what the center does and that she can call it in an emergency.

General Safety

- Once a child is thirteen, she can enroll in CPR and first-aid courses. Attend the class with your daughter.
- Repeat safety rules and knowledge often. Hearing it once is usually not enough.

Auto Safety

There is never an excuse for not wearing seat belts. Riding unrestrained greatly raises the risk for injury in car crashes.[16] Children under age twelve should also sit in the back seat, away from air bags, whenever possible.

When your adolescent daughter obtains her first driver's license or permit, establish rules and habits that will lay the groundwork for her safe driving habits. Parents need to be dedicated and vigilant to ensure that their children are properly trained to operate a vehicle safely. Statistics show that many teen drivers do not get adequate preparation or monitoring. Teens are also prone to more accidents due to reckless or aggressive behavior. Teens generally all mistakenly believe they can speed and still be safe.[17]

Facts

- Sixteen-year-olds have seven times as many car accidents as twenty-four-year-olds.
- Teen car accidents are more than two times as likely to be fatal or injury accidents.
- Teens speed more and wear seat belts less than adults.
- Teens get twice as many tickets as adults.
- Car crashes are the leading killer of teens in the United States.

Source: *Los Angeles Times,* May 18, 1997, Kathleen O. Ryan.

Since schools rarely teach driver's education anymore, the cost of private driving education can be expensive. Perhaps having your daughter pay for a portion of the education is a good way to impress upon her the seriousness of driving as a privilege. In most states, parents are not required to ride with their children who have earned a learner's permit. However, this practice is highly recommended and should be a rule in your family for as long as you believe your daughter needs supervision. Some states have graduated licensing programs that initially limit when a teen can drive and whether she can have passengers besides parents. This program then allows a teen to gradually earn more driving freedom. Consider what type of car your daughter will be driving. If at all possible look for the three Bs—big, belts, and bags.[18] Finally, watch your own driving. Parents who have more crashes and auto violations tend to have teens who have the most crashes and violations.

How to Help Your Child Become a Safe Driver

- Read the instruction manuals provided by your state licensing authority and by the driver instruction schools. Keep the manuals in the car.
- Practice first in large, empty parking lots at slow speeds. Next, move to wide empty roads.
- Teach your daughter that she should never assume that other drivers will drive safely and observe all traffic laws.
- Don't yell at your daughter while practicing. If you must, grab the wheel to steer or use the emergency brake.
- Relax and encourage your daughter.

Source: *Los Angeles Times*.

Questions to Ask Your Doctor

- My house was built in 1960. It has been repainted recently, but before that, lead paint was used. Should I have my child tested for lead?
- My daughter has been diagnosed as having a high blood level of lead. What is the treatment for this condition?
- What do you know about our city's water quality? Should I consider installing a water filter system or purchasing bottled water?
- My daughter has asthma. What can I do in the house to limit pollutants and minimize her risk?
- Is it safe for my child to play outdoors on days when the air quality is poor as long as she isn't running or playing hard?
- My daughter hates wearing her bicycle helmet and takes if off a lot. No amount of scolding seems to help. Will you discuss with her why she should wear her helmet?
- Do you think it is worth the cost of buying organic foods?

Resources

- Handgun Control, Inc., is a national citizens' group working to reduce gun violence. Call 310-446-0056 or visit www.handgun-control.org.
- For more information on protecting your child from lead, call the Alliance to End Childhood Lead Poisoning at 202-543-1147.
- For a brochure on lead in dishes contact the Environmental Defense Fund at 800-684-3322.
- The EPA's Safe Drinking Water Hotline can advise you on finding a lab to test your water. Call 800-426-4791.
- *Raising Children Toxic Free*, by Dr. Herbert L. Needleman and Dr. Philip J. Landrigan (Farrar, Straus and Giroux, 1994), is the definitive guide for parents on how you can protect children from toxic exposures and other environmental hazards.

- You can obtain information on air-polluting industries located near you by calling the EPA Community Right-to-Know hot line at 800-535-0202.
- For more information on lung health contact the American Lung Association, at 800-LUNG-USA or visit www.lungusa.org.
- A wonderful video that teaches children how to stay safe around dogs and cats is *Dogs, Cats & Kids: Learning to Be Safe with Animals*, moderated by Dr. Wayne Hunthausen (Donald Manelli & Associates, 1996).
- For information on reducing exposures that threaten our children join the Mothers & Others For a Livable Planet, 40 West Twentieth Street, New York, NY, 10011-4211. Call 888-ECO-INFO.
- The National SAFE Kids Campaign has information on a variety of safety topics. Call 202-662-0600.
- The Children's Health Environmental Coalition is a nonprofit organization that works to protect children's right to a safe environment. The organization distributes information and builds support for legislative initiatives that favor children. Call 310-589-2233.
- The National Coalition Against the Misuse of Pesticides is a nonprofit organization working to reduce the threat of pesticide use. Call 202-543-5450.

CHAPTER 20

Health Care: How to Get the Best for Your Daughter

"My mom told me one day, 'You're going to meet a new doctor.' When we got there, it was a guy. I'm like, I'm not going in there. I didn't want a guy looking at me. We went up front and asked the lady in charge for another doctor. They said, 'Oh, okay, we'll get you a female doctor.' So we went in, but I was so nervous. The doctor came in and said, 'Will you please take off your clothes? I'll be right back.' I'm like, oh my god. She said to put this robe on. I was so cold. Then she came in and said, 'Okay, you can lie down, I need to check your breasts.' I was like, oh my god, she's going to touch me. I'm a giggle person. When people touch me, I start laughing. She said, 'It's okay, you'll get used to it.' She asked me questions. If I had

sex. If somebody has ever touched me. My mom was right there,
so I was uncomfortable. But I just told her the truth."

—Katarina, age fifteen

AFTER the years of repeated ear infections, high fevers, and
strange rashes, you might find your daughter's middle childhood and teen years are something of a relief. To be sure, your
daughter probably won't have as many infectious illnesses or accidents that require stitches or X rays. Taking her to the doctor
once a year may seem, on the surface, like a waste of time and
money. Your daughter, too, may resist an annual physical. Both
children and adolescents generally do not see the need to visit a
doctor unless they have a problem.[1] Sharon has seen the years slip
by without taking her daughter, Caitlyn, sixteen, to the doctor.
"She will only go if she is really sick," says Sharon. "At about thirteen she started refusing to go if it was only for a checkup."

Thus, just when they need it the most, many girls fall into a
health care abyss. Don't allow this to happen to your daughter. As
we've seen in the preceding chapters, a lot of important changes
are still taking place in her body. And, as she enters the teen years,
your daughter will be making important decisions about smoking, nutrition, drug use, sexual activity, sports participation and
other issues that may affect her for her entire life.

In other words, the period from six to sixteen is no time to
stop seeing a doctor.

These are the years during which a health care professional
can help your daughter develop good preventive health habits
that will yield lifelong benefits. Going to the doctor faithfully
once a year will also help her understand that she has a responsibility to keep her body well by utilizing preventive health care.
An annual visit to the doctor serves to remind your daughter that
her health is a priority. The visit also promotes a relationship

between the doctor and the patient that may come in handy if sensitive health issues eventually arise. An annual preventive care visit doesn't mean a sports physical performed at school or sports camp. They are usually cursory and limited in scope.

Finding a Doctor

Besides the challenge of convincing your daughter to go to the doctor, you may struggle to find a health care provider who is sensitive to the many complex health issues that surround developing girls in our modern culture. A major dilemma is that girls become too old for the pediatrician and yet may feel too young for the ob-gyn. "I don't enjoy when they make you wear those white gowns because they leave the door partially open," says Ann-Marie, fifteen. "When I shut the door, there is still a large window. And when I try to change, all these little kids stare straight through the window and watch me change. It's unbearable because the doctors don't do anything about it. And they treat me like a baby."

Many teenage girls start feeling uncomfortable in a pediatrician's office. Kris experienced this with her sixteen-year-old, Tawny. "She really wanted to change doctors because she felt too old for a pediatrician. She hated sitting in a room full of toddlers and babies. Now, she hates sitting in a room with 'old' people in it!" Moreover, many girls are guarded, wary, embarrassed by, and mistrustful of doctors. Carla, fifteen, is nervous the minute the doctor walks into the room, says her mother, Delores. "She will not take her shirt off for him to check her heart or lungs. She is very uncomfortable with that, and I don't make her do it."

If you already have a pediatrician and your daughter is twelve or younger, you may want to stay with that doctor if he or she is someone you like and trust. If your daughter likes the doctor, but is starting to feel uncomfortable about the office (babyish decorations and a waiting room full of toddlers), ask the doctor if he or she sets aside special hours for older kids.

Once girls reach adolescence, finding the right doctor becomes more of an issue. You can stay with your pediatrician if the doctor says he or she is comfortable with adolescents and likes to treat them. One advantage of staying with a pediatrician is that teens are more likely to share information with a doctor they know and have seen regularly. Nina says her daughter, Keita, sixteen, has no qualms about seeing her pediatrician. "I thought she was too old for a pediatrician and a male doctor and suggested several possibilities. But she preferred to stay with her pediatrician, and he says she can come there as long as she wants." Pediatricians who treat teenagers, however, need to provide a full range of services for teens.[2] Not all pediatricians do this.

Another option is to take your daughter to an obstetrician-gynecologist. The Academy of Obstetricians and Gynecologists is working harder to reach out to adolescents and make them feel comfortable.[3] Still, your daughter may find it strange to sit in a waiting room with pregnant women. You may also worry that a visit to an ob-gyn means your daughter will have a pelvic exam. Discuss your concerns with the doctor prior to the examination. In general, ACOG advises that girls undergo a pelvic exam at age eighteen or earlier if a girl is sexually active. For sexually active girls, a pelvic exam every six months is sometimes recommended to check for STDs. Taking your daughter to an ob-gyn should not send a signal to your daughter that you expect her to be sexually active. You can explain to her that ob-gyns provide basic preventive care and are experts in menstruation and other female health issues. ACOG recommends that girls have their first ob-gyn visit for preventive services and screening at ages thirteen through fifteen. Teens benefit especially from seeing ob-gyns when they have menstrual abnormalities or unusual vaginal discharge.

Primary care doctors, internists, and family practitioners are also trained to see adolescents and provide a full range of preventive care and gynecological services. Finally, there is a small but growing number of doctors who specialize in adolescent medicine. These doctors are often women and typically work in designated teen clinics. However, there are only about 1,000 members of the Society for Adolescent Medicine.

While it's preferable that you accompany your daughter to a doctor's visit, your daughter should know that free clinics and school health clinics are other places where she can obtain medical care on her own initiative.

School-based clinics are convenient, comfortable, offer confidentiality, and are typically free. Many clinics, however, are limited in what they can provide. Clinics linked to a school but not actually on school property may be able to offer more services, such as dispensing birth control.

Free clinics are important alternatives to adolescents who don't want to involve their parents in health care decisions. Many free clinics are sensitive to teens and create comfortable environments in order to encourage patients to follow the professional advice and return for follow-up care. Planned Parenthood clinics are another good alternative for teens. While it is surely your desire to be involved in your daughter's health care, she should be informed about local clinics that will respect her desire for privacy and will treat her regardless of her ability to pay. In general, "teen friendly" health care facilities are nonjudgmental and respect teens regardless of their behaviors.[4] They offer free testing and a broad range of teen health services, including HIV testing. They honor confidentiality, are convenient, and require less paperwork and questions.

The Problem with Female Adolescent Health Care

"The teenage girl is almost no doctor's primary business."
—from *New York* magazine, February 8, 1999

While many doctors are supposedly qualified to treat adolescents, some of them don't do a very good job at it. This isn't all that surprising when you consider that even adult women often don't get thorough preventive care at their annual checkups unless their physician is up-to-date on all current issues and guidelines in women's health. Many women today are not asked about exercise or their relationships and may even not get a recommended screening test.[5] The situation is even worse for our daughters. Despite the acute need for girls—especially adolescents—to discuss their lifestyles and health-risk behaviors with doctors, few girls get good preventive care.[6] This fear has led Liv to look for a young doctor for her daughter Tara, fifteen. "If they were educated before 1990, I don't think many doctors keep up with current issues. And they are just not as sensitive as they could be."

In fact, doctors of all specialties are notoriously bad at dealing with issues that affect teens. Doctors are often at a loss over how to communicate with wary and guarded teens. They may avoid topics that are uncomfortable for them and their patients. One survey found that half of all doctors who treat adolescents do not discuss sex and sexual risk prevention, even though the high number of teens who are sexually active is well-recognized.[7] This is particularly sad in light of another part of the survey, which found that teens would trust doctors to keep their issues private—if only the doctor would ask.[8]

A survey of 2,026 high school students found that most doctors fail to ask students about important health issues.

Topic	Doctor and adolescent discussed it
Avoiding getting AIDS from sex	39%
Using condoms	37%
Adolescent's sex life	15%
How to say no to unwanted sex	13%
Sexual orientation	8%

Source: Mark A. Schuster, M.D., et al, "Communication Between Adolescents and Physicians About Sexual Behavior and Risk Prevention," *Archives of Pediatric and Adolescent Medicine*, Vol. 150, 1996.

Doctors who are interested in quality care for adolescents should be familiar with a government report called Guidelines for Preventive Care. It describes conditions that doctors should screen for and suggests that time be set aside to answer a teen's questions.

Not only should doctors who care for adolescents understand the vast range of health issues that confront teens, they should understand how to communicate with their young patients. Teens will resist getting care if they think the health care staff doesn't respect them or is judging them.[9] Consider attitude and treatment when finding a service provider for your daughter. Teens are hypersensitive and will be offended at negative attitudes from health care professionals. Raquel, sixteen, described her experience at a health clinic this way:[10] "The nurse kept asking me if I wanted to be pregnant. Like I'm ignorant, to belittle me because I'm young and I'm having sex. And I didn't feel that it was right, because at least I was responsible enough to use birth control and condoms and make sure I was all right, that I wasn't being hurt. I didn't like how they treated me."

While girls like Raquel will refuse to return to health care providers who insult them, girls tend to fully trust providers who offer a warm, caring atmosphere. Adolescents want to be able to talk to sensitive health care providers about issues that concern them. One survey found that two-thirds of girls wanted to discuss drugs, alcohol, smoking, eating disorders, STDs, abuse, and pregnancy prevention with their doctors.[11] But 35 percent of the girls said they were too embarrassed, afraid, or uncomfortable to discuss a problem with a doctor or health professional. Girls who were abused or depressed were the least likely to speak up about their problems. The survey also found that:

- About half of girls would prefer to have a female provider. Many girls say their preferences were stated but not met.
- Half of the younger girls and one-third of the older girls did not have an opportunity to speak privately with the doctor. One third would have preferred private time.

It's important to have a provider with whom your daughter feels comfortable, because, as she gets older, she may not want to tell you everything about her life. And few doctors who aren't specializing in adolescent medicine truly know how to make a girl comfortable enough to elicit important details about her health. Many girls typically talk more openly to women doctors.[12] Nina, whose older daughter wanted to stay with her pediatrician, discovered that her younger daughter, Antoinette, thirteen, wanted to see a woman doctor when her body began to change with the onset of puberty. "She wanted a woman doctor around age eleven, and we found one. She is a family friend." Many girls believe a woman will understand them better and will not patronize them. If your daughter sees a male practitioner and will be undergoing a pelvic exam, explain to her that a nurse will be present throughout the examination.

What Your Daughter Should Expect from a Health Care Provider in Virtually All Situations

- Be treated with respect. Never made to feel guilty, bad, or stupid.
- Empowerment. To feel in control of her body and remember that she is the ultimate decision-maker.
- Joint decision-making. To be able to work with the provider to make decisions.
- Education. To learn from the provider about her body and how to maintain good health.
- Confidentiality. That her discussions will not be revealed except in a life-threatening emergency.
- Trust. To be able to share freely what is bothering her.

Source: Dr. Alvin Goldfarb, executive director of the North American Society for Pediatric and Adolescent Gynecology.

Consent and Confidentiality Issues

Most parents begin to wonder when they should give their daughter more responsibility for her own health. That issue becomes pivotal when it comes to doctor's visits. Around the time of puberty, it is probably time for you to step out of the examination room and let your daughter have private time with the physician.[13] Some girls, however, feel too shy or uncomfortable with doctors to be alone. "She has the choice of whether I go in the exam room or not. But so far she refuses to let me leave her by herself," says Sharon, mother of sixteen-year-old Caitlyn. Another option is to remain in the room but leave at some point to give the doctor and your daughter time to talk privately. This will allow your daughter and the doctor to form a stronger relationship.

Both parents and their children should be familiar with two legal concepts that govern health care for minors. They are: consent and confidentiality. Consent and confidentiality laws vary by state. You should know the laws in your state regarding these issues, and your daughter should know them, too.

Consent: This law means that most children age fourteen and older can obtain medical care without a parent's permission, although these laws vary widely from state to state. Emergency care is always treated without consent although health care providers must try and reach a legal guardian. Nonemergency situations are more complex. Typically, however, a teenager can obtain nonemergency care, such as for treatment of a sexually transmitted disease or to obtain contraceptives. Most doctors honor a teen's request to provide care without parental permission because they understand that the teen probably would not seek the care if a parent had to be informed and would place themselves at risk for pregnancy or disease. Most states also allow pregnant teens to seek prenatal care without consent. STD testing is also widely available without consent.

Exceptions to this rule typically involve abortion and threat of suicide. Various states have laws requiring parental permission for treatment. Moreover, when a minor seeks treatment for abuse, the doctor is required to report the injuries to child protection authorities.

"My doctor is really nice, so I don't mind going. I can trust her, and she talks to me about stuff. Last time, she asked me if I was sexually active. I said no. My mom was standing next to me. A few minutes later, she told my mom to go out of the room, and she asked me again. I said no. She said, are you sure? I said I'm not. If I have questions about things, I feel I can ask her."

—Graciella, age sixteen

Confidentiality: Most health care providers want parents to be involved in their child's health care and medical treatment and will encourage children to involve their parents in decisions. However, if a teenager wants confidential treatment, it will typically be honored. This is an important area to some teenagers. Many would simply not seek care or preventive services if they were not guaranteed confidentiality. This fifteen-year-old girl who went to see her family's doctor put her concerns this way: "The doctor asked me questions like, 'Are you sexually active?' And I said, 'No.' I'm a little nervous, she knows my whole family . . . She would probably look at me differently."[14]

Doctors do not have to disclose sexual information to parents. If teens know this, they might be more willing to talk openly to a doctor. Doctors are not required by law to tell parents about a pregnancy, STD, or use of contraceptives.

While it may be hard for you as a parent to accept that your daughter might seek medical care without your involvement, remember that this alternative is far preferable to another option: That your daughter doesn't seek any care and puts herself at risk for disease or injury. Be assured that most health professionals encourage girls to notify their parents and tell them the truth.

Confidentiality is terribly important to some girls when it comes to getting needed medical care. Not wanting to tell parents of a health problem is a reason some girls don't get care when they need it. One survey found two in five teens cited this concern as a reason for avoiding needed health care.[16]

Cultural and Economic Considerations

Culturally sensitive care is very important to some girls. This includes speaking their language, understanding customs and beliefs, superstitions, patterns, and prevalence of disease in a particular ethnic group. Failure to understand cultural beliefs can lead to misdiagnosis, lack of cooperation, alienation of the patient from the health care system, and poor use of services.[17] It may be important for your daughter to see a provider of a like ethnicity or race. But remember that doesn't necessarily mean the person is a good listener.

Another major reason why too many girls do not get good health care is because they or their parents cannot afford it. All girls today are at risk for a myriad of significant health problems. Those who are poor are at even higher risk. More than one-quarter of high school girls said in one survey that they did not have access to health care when they needed it in the previous year.[18] As many as 44 percent of girls who were uninsured went without care when they needed it. About one-third of all uninsured girls lack a regular doctor.[19] If your family is uninsured and you cannot afford a private physician, look for a county or free health clinic and make regular appointments for your daughter. Check with your state department of health services to inquire about programs for free or low-cost health care for minors. Most states have such programs. Families who are residing in this country illegally can also obtain free health care without worrying about having their immigration status revealed. Finally, all caring parents should support political efforts to create a national system that provides quality health care to all minors regardless of ability to pay.

What Annual Exams Should Include

Annual medical exams for children and teens include the basics that patients of almost any age endure: a medical history, a physical exam (from head to toe), and lab tests.[18]

Children ages six to twelve should be checked for updated immunizations. This is important because new vaccines have been added with amazing frequency in the past five years, and

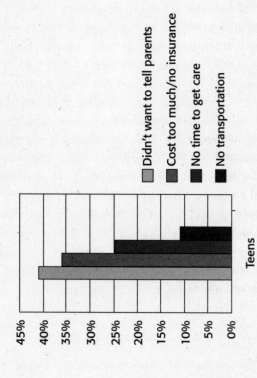

Why Girls Don't Get Health Care

Girls have many obstacles to obtaining health care, including their concern over privacy.

Teens

- ■ Didn't want to tell parents
- ■ Cost too much/no insurance
- ■ No time to get care
- ■ No transportation

45%
40%
35%
30%
25%
20%
15%
10%
5%
0%

Source: Commonwealth Fund.

your daughter may have missed something, such as the Varicella shot for preventing chicken pox or the Hepatitis B series of shots. Children ages six to twelve are also screened for tuberculosis, which is extremely important in large urban areas where active TB is a problem. Doctors should still inquire about a child's eating habits. And girls ten to twelve should be asked if they have any questions about their sexual development. The American Medical Association also recommends that doctors warn children in this age group about substance abuse and safety rules, like wearing bicycle helmets. Parents should be asked whether their child is having any problems in school, behavioral or learning related.

Girls thirteen to sixteen should spend more time with the doctor talking about social experiences, behaviors, and lifestyles that contribute to health. This includes a discussion of nutrition, exercise, and safety. Teens should be screened for the onset of several disorders or conditions, such as eating disorders, tuberculosis, dental problems, vision and hearing deficits, and scoliosis. Immunizations should be reviewed and updated. Teens should learn how to perform a monthly breast exam and should have the breasts examined by the doctor once a year. If a teen is sexually active, the doctor should perform a gynecological exam, Pap smear, and screen for STDs. Teens should be asked about behaviors that impact health, such as sexual activity, use of alcohol or other drugs, smoking habits, learning problems or difficulties in school, how to resolve personal conflicts without violence, the importance of exercise, and prevention of sports injuries. Finally, many health experts today suggest that children and teens be asked about their media habits, such as how often they watch TV and what they watch.

Not all of the responsibility for a thorough evaluation lies with the doctor. Your daughter should understand that she has to

A media history includes:

- How many hours a day do you watch television?
- How do you decide what shows to watch? Movies?
- Where is (are) the television(s)?
- Are there any house rules regarding viewing (e.g., no viewing until all homework is completed)?
- What are your favorite television programs? Movies?
- Are there rules regarding music videos? Video games?
- Who watches television with you?
- Do you surf the Internet?

contribute to the doctor's visit if it's to be successful. She should be encouraged to communicate openly with the doctor. This can take some time and practice. Barbara's sixteen-year-old daughter, Serena, is extremely withdrawn around her doctor and prefers that Barbara remain in the exam room. But Barbara tries to remain in the background—sometimes unsuccessfully. "She has always been encouraged to do 'the answering' when the doctor asks a question. But she still feels uncomfortable answering and sometimes will look at me with these pleading eyes to answer for her."

Questions to Ask Your Doctor

- What ages of children do you feel comfortable with?
- Do you have the time and the interest to discuss behavioral issues with my daughter, like media habits, sexual activity, and exercise habits?
- Do you see a girl alone or require that the parent be present?
- Do you keep current with research in adolescent medicine and guidelines for treatment?

- Can you refer me to a doctor who is very good at caring for adolescents?

Resources

- The Society for Adolescent Medicine provides names of health care providers. Call 816-224-8010.
- You can find a female doctor who specializes in seeing girls or adolescents by calling the American Medical Women's Association at 703-838-0500.
- The Adolescent Directory On-Line is an electronic guide to information on adolescent issues. It is operated by the Center for Adolescent Studies at the School of Education at Indiana University. Teens and parents can obtain information about a wide array of health issues. There is an inviting site for teens and a page to help teens and parents find counselors and health organizations. Visit www.education.indiana.edu/cas/adol/welcome.html.
- The American Academy of Pediatrics has a web page with detailed information about children's health care. Visit www.aap.org.
- The American Medical Association has greatly expanded its web pages, featuring information for consumers, including child health issues. Visit www.ama-assn.org.

Epilogue: A Healthy Family

REMEMBER how she felt, looked, smelled when she was a newborn? No doubt, as you cradled your baby daughter, you vowed to keep her as safe, healthy, and happy as you possibly could. As our children grow up, we often find that those goals aren't as easy as we'd imagined. Each family has its own strengths and weaknesses, each child her own propensity for brillance and harm. And, of course, some children are simply born with more opportunity for good health than others.

Whatever the circumstances, your daughter will thrive within a family that values being healthy, just like the individual flower that grows within a well-tended garden. Strive to keep your entire family in mind as you address goals that will benefit your daughter. Healthy families are ones that make special time together, to relax, play, and enjoy one another. They are families that establish rules for the safety of all. In healthy families, parents are available to answer questions and to listen with patience. Healthy families do not accept misbehavior, rudeness, violence, or abuse.

Your daughter will appreciate parents who set good examples, teach her how to care for herself, and be responsible for her choices. She will blossom in the embrace of a family that accepts her appearance, personality, talents, and limitations for what they are. A healthy family offers unconditional love.

A healthy family allows feelings to be shared. It does not judge the actions of others but offers guidance and forgiveness. A healthy family is a secure one.

Helping your daughter grow up healthy is a process that begins in that place deep within your heart.

"There is no creature whose inward being is so strong that it is not greatly determined by what lies outside of it."

—George Eliot

Chapter Notes

Chapter 1: Introduction

1. "The author of a 1999 report . . ." Susan Brenna, "The Silent Treatment," *New York* magazine, February 8, 1999.
2. "In 1998, the American . . ." Dr. Paula Hillard, remarks made at the American College of Obstetricians and Gynecologists Committee on Adolescent Health Care, 1998.
3. "Fifty-eight percent of girls . . ." The Commonwealth Fund Survey on the Health of Adolescent Girls, November 1997.
4. "One in six girls . . ." Commonwealth Fund.
5. "One in four . . ." U.S. Centers for Disease Control and Prevention.
6. "Twenty-five percent of girls say . . ." Commonwealth Fund.
7. "Sixty-six percent of girls have . . ." American College of Obstetricians and Gynecologists (ACOG) Committee on Adolescent Health Care, 1998.
8. "Four in ten teens . . ." ACOG.
9. "One in five U.S. . . ." ACOG.
10. "Eighty-five percent of girls . . ." ACOG.
11. "Thirty-four percent of high school . . ." ACOG.
12. "Fifteen percent of high school . . ." ACOG.
13. "Eighteen percent of high school . . ." ACOG.
14. "Twenty-two percent of high school . . ." ACOG.
15. "One in four . . ." ACOG.
16. "Half of all new . . ." U.S. Department of Health and Human Services (HHS).

17. "Three million teens . . ." HHS; ACOG.

18. "Twenty-five of American . . ." Associated Press, "Youth Health Still Declining in America, Study Says," June 7, 1995, on research by Dr. Michelle Wilson in the *Journal of the American Medical Association.*

19. "Suicide rates among . . ." KidsPeace Survey, The National Center for Kids in Crisis, May 10, 1995.

20. "Forty percent of American . . ." President's Council on Physical Fitness and Sports, 1994.

21. "Forty-three percent of kids live . . ." *Prevention* Children's Health Index, 1995.

22. "Sixteen percent of children . . ." *Prevention.*

23. "The ten- to nineteen- . . ." David and Lucile Packard Foundation, "The Future of Children," 1992.

24. "A survey by . . ." Prevention Children's Health Index, 1995.

25. "By 1990, more than . . ." Carnegie Corporation of America report, "A Developmental Strategy to Prevent Lifelong Damage," 1995.

26. "According to one . . ." Michael D. Resnick, et al., "Close Ties to Parents, School Improve Adolescents' Lives," *Minnesota Medicine*, Vol. 80, No. 2, December 1997.

27. "Girls today are . . ." The National Council for Research on Women, "The Girls Report: What We Know and Need to Know about Growing Up Female," 1998.

28. "The Carnegie Corporation report . . ." Carnegie Corporation.

29. "And, at the 1997 . . ." Richard P. Dukes, et al.; Diana P. Oliver, et al.; and Dale Kunkel, et al.; remarks made at the annual American Psychological Association meeting, August 15, 1997.

30. "One study of . . ." Richard Jessor, et al., "Protective Factors in Adolescent Health Behavior," *Journal of Personality and Social Psychology*, Vol. 75, No. 3, 1998.

31. "A landmark 1997 . . ." Michael D. Resnick, et al.

32. "Research has concluded . . ." K. A. S. Wickrama, et al.; "The Intergenerational Transmission of Health-Risk Behaviors: Adolescent Lifestyles and Gender-Moderating Effects," *Journal of Health and Social Behavior*, Vol. 40, No. 3, September 1999.

33. "A window of opportunity . . ." Kaiser Family Foundation survey, 1991.

34. "You have a real feeling . . ." Remarks by Matt James, president, Kaiser

Family Foundation, made March 1, 1999, Los Angeles, press conference on "Talking with Kids about Tough Issues."

Chapter 2: Bones

1. "There is also some . . ." Deborah A. Galuska and Maryfran R. Sowers, "Menstrual History and Bone Density in Young Women," *Journal of Women's Health and Gender-Specific Medicine*, Vol. 8, No. 5, 1999.
2. "Moreover some families . . ." Baylor University press release on research by Steven Abram, July 2, 1999.
3. "In particular, some people . . ." Terence Momaney, *Los Angeles Times*, July 10, 1997, "Osteoporosis Clues Found in Research on Girls' Genes." On research published in the *New England Journal of Medicine*.
4. "Forty-five percent . . ." American Academy of Orthopaedic Surgeons press release, October 21, 1995. Remarks by Dr. Laura Tosi.
5. "What this means is . . ." Ohio State University press release, May 31, 1995. Research by Gordon Wardlaw, et al.
6. "In 1997, the National . . ." A more recent policy statement on calcium requirements in children and adolescents was released by American Academy of Pediatrics Committee on Nutrition in the journal *Pediatrics*, vol. 104, No. 5, November 1999. The statement supported recommendations for 1,200 to 1,500 mg calcium for girls beginning in the preteen years and continuing through adolescence.
7. "More than eight out . . ." Reuters, January 28, 1999, "Nutritionists Develop Website so Teens Get Milk."
8. "Most girls consume . . ." United States Deptartment of Agriculture.
9. "And the years just before . . ." Dr. Karl Insogna, et al., "Boning Up on Osteoporosis: What's New?" *Journal of Women's Health*, Vol. 8, No. 5, 1999.
10. "Studies show the spines . . ." National Dairy Council press release, 1996.
11. "Some girls may think . . ." ibid.
12. "The young women . . ." Purdue University press release, August 1996, on research by Dorothy Teegarden.
13. "A modest increase . . ." National Dairy Council, 1996, from research first reported in *Pediatrics*.
14. "Bone, like muscle . . ." American Academy of Orthopaedic Surgeons.

15. "One study found that . . ." Ohio State University press release, October 31, 1996, on research by Jasmika K. Ilich, et al.
16. "One poll of girls . . ." National Dairy Council.
17. "Experts call milk . . ." American Academy of Orthopaedic Surgeons.
18. "But teens may actually . . ." *Dairy Council Digest*, Vol. 67, No. 3, May/June 1996.
19. "The more sodium . . ." Ohio State University.
20. "Two-thirds of girls . . ." National Dairy Council.
21. "One in four teens . . ." National Dairy Council on research published in the *Journal of Adolescent Health*.

Chapter 3: Skin Care

1. "Eighty percent of an . . ." American Academy of Dermatology, "Skin Savvy" campaign, 1998.
2. "Even one or two . . ." Karen Glanz, Ph.D., "Participation, Retention, and Adherence: Implications for Health Promotion Research and Practice [comment]," *Journal of Health Education and Behavior*, Vol. 13, No. 5, May/June 1999.
3. "But less than half . . ." ibid.
4. "And sunscreen alone . . ." American Cancer Society; presented at the Society for Epidemiological Research in Baltimore, June, 16, 1999.
5. "According to health . . ." American Academy of Dermatology web site, 1999.
6. "Astonishingly, surveys find . . ." Shari Roan, "Suffering in Silence," *Los Angeles Times*, January 10, 1995, on remarks by Dr. Diane Baker.
7. "I think the . . ." ibid.
8. "Acne occurs in . . ." ibid.
9. "Five percent of all . . ." ibid.
10. "It often takes . . ." ibid.
11. "Serious complications from . . ." Shari Roan, "The Problems with Piercings," *Los Angeles Times*, November 21, 1995.
12. "Nickel in inexpensive . . ." American Academy of Dermatology.
13. "Nickel allergies have . . ." ibid.
14. "About 10 percent of all . . ." ibid.

Chapter 4: Body Image and Self-esteem

1. "The number of girls . . ." Mark Moran, *American Medical News*, October 26, 1998.

2. "These girls will do . . ." Joan Jacobs Blumberg, *The Body Project: An Intimate History of American Girls*, Random House, 1997.

3. "A study looking at . . ." Mimi Nichter, et al., "Hype and Weight," Medical *Anthropology*, Vol. 13, No. 3, September 1991.

4. "There appears to be . . ." Carol Gilligan, *In a Different Voice*, Harvard University Press, 1982.

5. "So common is . . ." Jennifer Read, "Body Dissatisfaction as a Development Stage in Preadolescent Girls," paper presented at the American Psychological Association meeting, 1994.

6. "Some girls as young . . ." Dr. Dean Krahn, presented at the American Psychiatric Association meeting, May 25, 1995. The study, from psychiatrists at the University of Wisconsin, found evidence that children who diet during their preteen years may be more likely than other children to use alcohol and cigarettes once they become adolescents.

7. "One study found that . . ." Marnell Jameson, "Mothers, Daughters and Weight," *Los Angeles Times*, September 22, 1996, reporting on research by Adam Drewnowski, a professor of public health at the University of Michigan, who studied 2,000 girls ages eleven to eighteen and 1,300 mothers. In another study by Rebecca Manley of the Massachusetts Eating Disorders Foundation, girls not only dieted because their mothers did but also internalized their mother's complaints about her own body, such as "I hate my thighs" or "I look so fat."

8. "In one study, more than 70 percent . . ." Mimi Nichter, et al., "Body Image and Weight Concerns Among African-American and White Adolescent Females: Differences Which Makes a Difference." Presented in 1993.

9. "Dieting itself, according . . ." Simone A. French, Ph.D., et al., "Frequent Dieting Among Adolescents," *American Journal of Public Health*, Vol. 85, No. 5, May 1995, French's study of 33,393 Minnesota students in grades seven through twelve found that 85 percent of the girls who said they never dieted reported a positive body image compared with 34.7 percent who said they always dieted.

10. "Girls who diet . . ." ibid.

11. "The average child spends . . ." Richard Kahlenberg, "V-Chipping Away at Unhealthy Television," *Los Angeles Times*, January 18, 1996.

12. "One study found up to . . ." Lynn Smith, "Family Hour Provides No Haven From Sexual Messages," *Los Angeles Times*, Dec. 29, 1996.

13. "The more girls dwelled . . ." Alison E. Field, et al., "Relation of Peer and Media Influences to the Development of Purging Behaviors Among Preadolescent and Adolescent Girls," *Archives of Pediatric and Adolescent Medicine*, Vol. 53, No. 11, November 1999.

14. "Girls, in particular . . ." Children Now, 1996 survey.

15. "Religious affiliation and . . ." Christopher G. Ellison, et al., "Public Health and Health Education in Faith Communities," *Health Education & Behavior Journal*, October 1998.

Chapter 5: Fitness and Weight Control

1. "Obesity affects one . . ." Dr. William Dietz, "The causes and health consequences of obesity in children and adolescents," *Pediatrics*, Vol. 101, No. 3, March 1998.

2. "Surveys show that . . ." *Patient Care*, October 15, 1998.

3. "Today we know . . ." Frances M. Berg, *Afraid to Eat: Children and Teens in Weight Crisis*, Healthy Weight Publishing Network, 1997.

4. "One study found . . ." Nicole Evans, et al., "Adolescents' Perceptions of Their Peers' Health Norms," *American Journal of Public Health*, Vol. 85, No. 8, August 1995.

5. "In a 1992 survey . . ." L. Kann, *Morbidity and Mortality Report*, Vol. 44, 1995.

6. "Studies show, however . . ." Berg.

7. "A study of eighty-three . . ." Wendy Roncolato and Gail Huon, presented at a meeting of the British Psychological Society, April 3, 1997.

8. "When children are . . ." Claude Bouchard, M.D., "Physical Activity, Genetic and Nutritional Considerations in Childhood Weight Management," American College of Sports Medicine conference, July 16, 1996.

9. "And, in about . . ." Bouchard.

10. "As many as 45 percent . . ." K. S. Tippet, et al., "Food and Nutrition Intakes by Individuals in the U.S., One Day," 1989–91 Nationwide Food Survey, No. 91–2, September 1995.

11. "One survey found . . ." International Life Sciences Institute report *Improving Children's Health through Physical Activity*, July 1997.

12. "A 1998 study . . ." Ross Anderson, Ph.D., American Council on Exercise, August. 27, 1998.

13. "One fascinating study . . ." Thomas N. Robinson, presented at a meeting of the Pediatric Academic Societies, May 4, 1999.

14. "A typical child . . ." American College of Sports Medicine conference, July 16, 1996.

15. "Obese children, it . . ." Ginger Thompson, "With Obesity in Children Rising, More Get Adult Type of Diabetes," *New York Times*, December 13, 1998.

16. "Obese children do . . ." William Dietz, M.D., "The causes and health consequences of obesity in children and adolescents," *Pediatrics*, Vol. 101, No. 3, March 1998.

17. "Weight loss programs . . ." Berg.

18. "Some weight-control," *Patient Care*, October. 15, 1998.

19. "According to the . . ." Council on Exercise press release, August 27, 1998.

20. "According to several . . ." The Fitness Products Council, "Tracking the Fitness Movement," 1996.

21. "Sedentary behavior in . . ." Russel Pate, "Associations between Physical Activity and Other Health Behaviors in a Representative Sample of U.S. Adolescents," *American Journal of Public Health*, Vol. 86, No. 11, November 1996.

22. "In 1994, the . . ." Dr. Rose Frisch, "Former Athletes Have a Lower Lifetime Occurrence of Breast Cancer and Cancers of the Reproductive System," *Adv. Exp. Medical Biology*, Vol. 322, 1992.

23. "One survey found . . ." Gallup survey conducted for the American Dietetic Association, President's Council, International Food Information Council, 1994.

24. "Children (especially) . . ." Harold W. Kohl III, Ph.D., and Karen E. Hobbs, *Pediatrics* Supplement, "The Causes and Health Consequences in Children and Adolescents," Vol. 101, No. 3, Part 2, March 1998.

25. "FACT: Parents can't . . ." American College of Sports Medicine and National Dairy Council Scientific Roundtable "Physical Activity, Genetic and Nutritional Considerations in Childhood Weight Management," July 24, 1996.

26. "And according to one . . ." ILSI 1997 poll.

27. "There's nothing wrong . . ." Pate.

28. "You have to purposefully . . ." Dr. Laura Walther Nathanson, *The Portable Pediatrician's Guide to Kids*, HarperPerennial, 1996.

Chapter 6: Sports and Athletics

1. "Girls account for . . ." President's Council on Physical Fitness and Sports report *Physical Activity and Sport in the Lives of Girls*, Spring 1997.

2. "And many studies have . . ." R. M. Page, et al., "Is School Sports Participation a Protective Factor Against Adolescent Health Risk Behaviors," *Journal of Health Education*, Vol. 29, May/June 1998. More documentation can be found in the U.S. Department of Health and Human Service's Girl Power public health campaign.

3. "In fact, a survey of . . ." Elizabeth Weil, "Good Sports," *Los Angeles Times*, January 2, 1996.

4. "Despite the clear advantage . . ." The Fitness Products Council, Sporting Goods Manufacturers' Association, *Tracking the Fitness Movement*, 1996.

5. "Starting young appears . . ." Melissa B. Tamberg, "Give Girls a Sporting Chance," *Parenting* magazine, March 1998.

6. "If a person has . . ." *Penn State Sports Medicine Newsletter* press release, October 20, 1997, on research by A. Eugene Coleman.

7. "Moreover, in some schools . . ." Jane Gottesman, "Is Cheerleading a Sneaky Way Around Title IX?" *The New York Times*, October 23, 1994.

8. "Many poor girls . . ." President's Council on Physical Fitness and Sports.

9. "The big negative in . . ." Weil.

10. "Another reason older . . ." The National Council for Research on Women, *The Girls Report*, 1998.

11. "Increasingly, athletic participation . . ." President's Council on Physical Fitness and Sports, *Physical Activity and Sport in the Lives of Girls*, Spring 1997.

12. "Girls who participate . . ." Beth Azar, "Public Scrutiny Sparks Some Eating Disorders," American Psychological Association, *Monitor*, July 1996, reporting on research by Donald Williamson, Ph.D., at Louisiana State University.

13. "About 775,000 kids . . ." U.S. Consumer Product Safety Commission.

14. "Injuries are most likely . . ." Sally S. Harris, M.D., remarks at the American College of Sports Medicine Scientific Roundtable on "Youth Sports Injury," November 5, 1996.

15. "Girls are particularly . . ." ibid.

16. "Girls may be at . . ." ibid.

17. "Strength training has . . ." American College of Sports Medicine "Current Comment," March 1998.

18. "As the number of . . ." William E. Garrett Jr., M.D., remarks made at the American Academy of Orthopaedic Surgeons Sixty-sixth Annual Meeting, Feb. 5, 1999.

19. "Females—especially those in . . ." ibid.

20. "Steroid use among girls . . ." Gary Legwold, "More Teenage Girls Using Steroids," *Better Homes & Gardens*, August 1998.

21. "They may cause heart . . ." ibid.

Chapter 7: Nutrition

1. "A lot of parents . . ." Bill Viand, M.D., personal interview, 1999.

2. "Studies show that . . ." Teresa A. Nicklas, Ph.D., "Impact of Breakfast Consumption on Nutritional Adequacy of the Diets of Young Adults in Bogalusa, Louisiana, Ethnic and Gender Contrasts," *Journal of the American Dietetic Association*, Vol. 98, No. 12, December 1998.

3. "More than 75 percent . . ." ibid.

4. "Children should be allowed . . ." International Food Information Council, IFIC web site, featuring remarks by Susan L. Johnson of the University of Colorado Center for Human Nutrition.

5. "One survey found that . . ." Janet Bode, *Food Fight: A Guide to Eating Disorders for Preteens and Their Parents*, Simon & Schuster, 1997.

6. "Planning is the key . . ." American Dietetic Association press release, July 15, 1998, remarks by Tammy Baker.

7. "Kids who eat a . . ." Ernesto Pollitt, Ph.D., "Does Breakfast Make a Difference in School?" *Journal of the American Dietetic Association*, Vol. 95, No. 10, October 1995.

8. "Children who do not . . ." American Heart Association "Health Fest" campaign materials, September 1997.

9. "Parents who impose . . ." Penn State University press release, November 8, 1994, on research by Susan Johnson and Leann Birch.

10. "Some children learn control . . ." ibid.

11. "For example, many . . ." Mattel Foundation, "Helping Kids Grow," 1994.

12. "Many young children are picky . . ." William H. Dietz, M.D., and Loraine Stern, M.D., *American Academy of Pediatrics Guide to Your Child's Nutrition*, Villard, 1998.

13. "More children today . . ." Department of Agriculture press release,

"What and where our children eat—1994 Nationwide Survey," April 18, 1996.

14. "Kids ages six . . ." ibid.

15. "Adolescents typically eat . . ." *Dairy Council Digest*, Vol. 67, No. 3, May/June 1996.

16. "Teens might even see . . ." ibid.

17. "As children near adulthood . . ." Nicklas.

18. "In an eye-opening survey . . ." Lucy B. Adams, "An Overview of Adolescent Eating Behaviors," *Annals of the New York Academy of Sciences*, Vol. 817, May 1997.

19. "Follow this rule of . . ." Christine L. Williams, M.D., "Is a High-Fiber Diet Safe for Children?" *Pediatrics*, Vol. 96, No.5, Part 2, November 1995.

20. "An estimated 25 percent . . ." Betsy Lozoff, M.D., remarks made at American Pediatric Societies meeting, Washington, D.C., May 5, 1997.

21. "Iron deficiency in . . ." ibid.

22. "The lack of iron . . ." *The Brown University Child and Adolescent Behavior Letter*, "Keep Your Eye on Iron Supplements," Vol. 11., No. 6, June 1995.

23. "One study found that . . ." *Nutrition Alert*, "Thinking About Iron," Vol. 3, No. 1, January /February, 1997.

24. "During periods of . . ." Dietz and Stern.

Chapter 8: Eating Disorders

1. "Victims of eating . . ." Richard E. Kreipe, M.D., "Eating Disorders Among Children and Adolescents," *Pediatrics in Review*, Vol. 16, No. 10, October 1995.

2. "In recent years . . ." Sue A. Kuba, Ph.D., and Diane J. Harris, Ph.D., "Ethnic Identity, Acculturation and Eating Disorders for Women of Color," presented at the Women's Health Conference, November 10, 1993.

3. "Sexual or physical abuse . . ." Rachel Bryant-Wagh and Bryan Lask, "Annotation: Eating Disorders in Childhood," *Journal of Child Psychology and Psychiatry*, Vol. 36, No. 2, 1998.

4. "Another study suggested . . ." Dianne Neumark-Sztainer, Ph.D., et al., "Body dissatisfaction and unhealthy weight control practices among adolescents with and without chronic illness: a population-based

study," *Archives of Pediatric and Adolescent Medicine*, Vol. 149, No. 12, December 1995.

5. "According to one study . . ." Frances M. Berg, *Afraid to Eat*, Healthy Weight Publishing, 1997.

6. "Experts usually use . . ." American Psychiatric Association *Diagnostic and Statistical Manual of Mental Disorders*, Fourth Edition, 1994.

7. "The disorder usually surfaces . . ." *Scientific American*, Explorations, Treatment of Eating Disorders, March 2, 1998.

8. "Researchers estimate that . . ." ibid.

9. "As many as 75 percent . . ." Kreipe.

10. "As Wisconsin therapist . . ." Ellyn M. Satter, "Childhood Eating Disorders," *Journal of the American Dietetic Association*, Vol. 86, No. 3, March 1986.

11. "About 40 percent of . . ." Kreipe.

12. "About 5 percent to 18 percent . . ." *Scientific American*.

13. "Bulimia is actually . . ." Berg.

14. "Symptoms of bulimia . . ." *Scientific American*.

15. "Bulimics are typically . . ." Kreipe.

16. "To diagnose the disorder . . ." *DSM*.

17. "Other signs of . . ." Berg.

18. "About 30 percent of people . . ." *Scientific American*.

19. "In 1995, medical experts . . ." Society for Adolescent Medicine press release, June 26, 1995.

20. "One study found that . . ." Ohio State University press release, August 17, 1997.

21. "In fact, an estimated . . ." Kreipe.

22. "Eating disorders are often . . ." Kreipe.

23. "And, according to one . . ." Lucy B. Adams and Mary-Ann B. Shafer, M.D., "Early Manifestations of Eating Disorders in Adolescents: Defining Those at Risk," *Journal of Nutrition Education*, Vol. 20, No. 6, 1988.

24. "It is often difficult . . ." ibid.

25. "Warning signs for . . ." ibid.

26. "Tips to prevent . . ." ibid.

Chapter 9: Preventing Major Diseases

1. "One in eight women . . ." American Heart Association, "The Difference in a Woman's Heart" campaign, 1994.

2. "Almost 14 million girls . . ." American Heart Association.

3. "Children with fat bellies . . ." Stephen R. Daniels, M.D., "Association of body fat distribution and cardiovascular risk factors in children and adolescents," *Circulation*, Vol. 99, No. 4, February 1999.

4. "One study of 7,000 . . ." Marilyn Winkleby, M.D., "Ethnic Variation in cardiovascular disease risk factors among children and young adults," *Journal of the American Medical Association*, Vol. 281, No. 11, March 17, 1999.

5. "For example, women who . . ." Meir Stampfer, M.D., remarks made at the American Heart Association annual meeting, November 9, 1999.

6. "Girls in grades three . . ." University of California, San Diego, press release on research by Philip R. Nader, M.D., July 14, 1999.

7. "If the problem surfaces . . ." Weihang Bao, et al., "Essential Hypertension Predicted by Tracking of Elevated Blood Pressure From Childhood to Adulthood," *American Journal of Hypertension*, Vol. 8, No. 7, July 1995.

8. "There is also strong . . ." Leena Taittonen, et al., "Angiotensin converting enzyme gene insertion/deletion polymorphism, angiotensinogen gene polymorphisms, family history of hypertension, and childhood blood pressure," *American Journal of Hypertension,* Vol. 12, No. 9, Part 1, September 1999.

9. "With the new guidelines . . ." National Heart, Lung and Blood Institute communications office, October 7, 1996.

10. "However, adolescent girls with . . ." ibid.

11. "According to the American . . ." American Academy of Pediatrics, "Where We Stand," October 1996.

12. "Children with confirmed . . ." American Heart Association press release, November 1994.

13. "Lung cancer is . . ." American Cancer Society, 1994.

14. "Smoking also increases . . ." ACS.

15. "The more cigarettes . . ." ACS.

16. "But there are strategies . . ." National Cancer Institute, Surveillance, Epidemiology and End Results Program, 1997.

17. "While studies have found . . ." Malcom Ritter, "Low-Fat Diet Won't Help the Middle-aged Avoid Breast Cancer," Associated Press, February 7, 1996.

18. "It is also abundantly . . ." C. L. Carpenter, et al., "Lifetime Exercise Activity and Breast Cancer Risk among Postmenopausal Women,"

British Journal of Cancer, Vol. 80, No. 11, August 1999. In addition, Beverly Rockhill reported in the *Archives of Internal Medicine* that women who exercise an hour a day reduce their breast cancer risk by 20 percent.

19. "Before leaving for college . . ." Carole G. Vogel, *Will I Get Breast Cancer?*, Julian Messner, 1995.

20. "If your daughter . . ." American Cancer Society press release "Talcum Powder and Cancer," February 17, 1998.

21. "About 15,000 U.S. . . ." American Medical Women's Association, "Global Solutions in Cervical Cancer" conference, February 1999.

22. "HPV affects 13 percent to . . ." Sharon M. Mount, M.D, and Jacalyn L. Papillo, "A Study of 10,246 Pediatric and Adolescent Papanicolaou Smear Diagnoses in Northern New England," *Pediatrics,* Vol. 103, No. 3, March 1999.

23. "Cervical cell abnormalities . . ." ibid.

24. "One study found . . ." National Cervical Cancer Public Education Campaign, American Medical Women's Association, January 1999.

25. "White or fair skinned . . ." "Detecting Skin Cancer," Patient Page, *Journal of the American Medical Association*, Vol. 281, No. 7, February 17, 1999.

26. "Any of these symptoms . . ." Donald F. Phillips, "New Insights into Endometriosis and Polycystic Ovary Syndrome," *Journal of the American Medical Association*, Vol. 280, No. 22, December 9, 1998.

27. "About 3 percent of girls . . ." "Urinary Tract Infections In Childhood," National Institute of Diabetes and Digestive and Kidney Disease, NIH Publication No. 97-4246, July 1997.

28. "The message for parents . . ." A. Barry Belman, M.D., remarks made at the Fifth Women's Health Congress, June 21, 1998.

29. "Nevertheless, if you want . . ." Laura J. Romanzi, M.D., "Urinary Incontinence: A Family Affair," *Journal of Gender Specific Medicine*, Vol. 1, No. 2, October/November 1998.

Chapter 10: Genetics

1. "Another downside to testing . . ." from the Health Insurance Portability Act.

2. "To help parents . . ." American Society of Human Genetics and the American College of Medical Genetics, "Points to Consider: Legal,

Ethical and Psychosocial Implications of Genetic Testing in Children and Adolescents," 1995.

3. "But scientists do . . ." Darrell E. Ward, "To know or not to know," Ohio State University James Cancer Hospital and Solóre Research Institute, *Frontiers*, Vol. 6, No. 2, Winter 1999.

4. "But the BRCA genes . . ." ibid.

5. "A granddaughter of someone . . ." ibid.

6. "If the gene is present . . ." Ellen Michaud, "Outsmart Your Bad Genes," *Prevention* magazine, April 1999.

Chapter 11: Reproductive Health

1. "The Sexuality Information . . ." The Sexuality Information and Education Council, "Talking About Sex," 1992.

2. "Kids can act rebellious . . ." American Social Health Association, "Becoming an Askable Parent," 1994.

3. "While your daughter . . ." Kaiser Family Foundation, "Survey on Teens and Sex," June 24, 1996.

4. "Many surveys in . . ." ibid.

5. "Their fascination with sexual . . ." Jane Brown, University of North Carolina, remarks made at Kaiser Family Foundation conference "Sex on TV," February 9, 1999.

6. "Kids whose mothers talked . . ." ibid.

7. "One million teenagers . . ." Alan Guttmacher Institute, 1998.

8. "One in five girls . . ." AGI, 1994.

9. "STDs . . ." Planned Parenthood Federation of America, Inc., 1996.

10. "In a single act . . ." PPF

11. "Females are much more . . ." AGI, Kaiser Family Foundation, "Emerging Issues in Reproductive Health," National Press Foundation, November 20, 1996.

12. "Females with STDs . . ." ibid.

13. "Teens are more likely . . ." ibid.

14. "Teenage girls are more . . ." AGI, PPF, "Sexual Behavior Among U.S. High School Students, 1990–1995," *Family Planning Perspectives*, July/August 1998.

15. "When females get STDs . . ." Emerging Issues.

16. "An estimated 15 percent . . ." ibid.

17. "For example, the number . . ." *Family Planning Perspectives.*

18. "Increasingly, the idea of . . ." Kaiser Family Foundation, National Survey of Teens, June 24, 1996.

19. "In one survey of . . ." ibid.

20. "Dr. Drew Pinksy . . ." Remarks made at KFF "Sex on TV" conference.

21. "In her book . . ." Wendy Shalit, *A Return to Modesty*, Free Press, 1999.

22. "Research has shown . . ." KFF, June 1996, survey.

23. "Teens who drink alcohol . . ." Karen L. Graves and Barbara C. Leigh, "The relationships of substance use to sexual activity among young adults in the United States," *Family Planning Perspectives*, Vol. 27, No. 1, January/February 1998.

24. "Girls whose family . . ." Steven Stack, "The Effect of Geographic Mobility on Premarital Sex," *Journal of Marriage and the Family,* Vol. 56, February 1994.

25. "For example, federal . . ." Gale Burstein, M.D., "Incident Chlamydia Tractomatis Infections Among Inner-city Adolescent Females," *Journal of the American Medical Association*, Vol. 280, No. 6, August 12, 1998.

26. "A survey found that . . ." Kaiser Family Foundation, Survey on HIV, 1998.

Chapter 12: Preadolescence

1. "A mother and her . . ." Robert Haber, M.D., "On Developmental Milestones," *Pediatrics*, Vol. 102, No. 4, October 1998.

2. "It used to be . . ." Paul Kaplowitz, M.D., "Redefining the age at which puberty is precocious in girls in the United States," *Pediatrics*, Vol. 104, No. 4, Part 1, October 1999.

3. "Girls who begin . . ." Darrell M. Wilson, M.D., "Timing and rate of sexual maturation and the onset of cigarette and alcohol use among teenage girls," *Archives of Pediatric and Adolescent Medicine*, Vol. 148, No. 8, August 1994.

4. "Children who look . . ." Trish Hall, "Moms and Daughters: Too Close for Comfort," *New York Times*, June 21, 1998.

5. "Studies show that . . ." ibid.

6. "Styles of dress and . . ." The Sexuality Information and Education Council, "Now What Do I Do? How to Give your Preteens Your Messages," 1996.

7. "In fourth or fifth . . ." Sara Estroff Marano, "Puberty May Start at 6 as Hormones Surge," *The New York Times*, July 1, 1997.

8. "Studies show that . . ." KidsPeace.
9. "Around age thirteen . . ." ibid.
10. "One study found . . ." ibid.

Chapter 13: Adolescence

1. "While the preteen years . . ." Dianne Hales, *Just Like A Woman: How Gender Science is Redefining What Makes Us Female*, Bantam Books, 1999.
2. "For girls who . . ." "Being adopted may not pose a problem until adolescence," *Brown University Child and Adolescent Behavior Letter*, 1998.
3. "One estimate suggested . . ." University of Illinois press release on research by Reed Larson, October 1996.
4. "Girls who are . . ." Ms. Foundation for Women, *Girls Seen and Heard: 52 Life Lessons for Our Daughters*, Jeremy P. Tarcher/Putnam, 1998.
5. "Girls who are living . . ." Lila A. Wallis, M.D., with Marian Betancourt, *The Whole Woman*, Avon Books, 1999.
6. "Teenage girls who . . ." The National Council for Research on Women, *The Girls Report*, 1998.
7. "In 1994, the brilliant . . ." Mary Pipher, *Reviving Ophelia: Saving the Selves of Adolescent Girls*, G. P. Putnam, 1994.
8. "This study found that . . ." National Campaign to Prevent Teenage Pregnancy, "Peer Potential: Making the Most of How Teens Influence Each Other," 1999.
9. "Many parents, and even . . ." National Sleep Foundation, August 19, 1999.
10. "About 23 percent of teenagers . . ." National Sleep Foundation 1999 Nationwide Omnibus Survey, September 27, 1999.

Chapter 14: Mental Health

1. "In all likelihood . . ." Katharine Davis Fishman, *Behind the One-Way Mirror: Psychotherapy and Children*, Bantam Books, 1995.
2. "And the rate of . . ." Hales, *Just Like a Woman*.
3. "And, like adults, negative . . ." Girls Inc., "Stress in the Lives of Adolescent Girls," December 1993.
4. "Because girls are socialized . . ." Judith V. Jordan, et al., *Women's Growth in Connection*, The Guilford Press, 1991.

5. "Divorce is one . . ." Karen D. Rudolph and Constance Hammer, "Age and gender as determinants of stress exposure, generation, and reactions in youngsters," *Child Development*, Vol. 70, No. 3, May/June 1999.

6. "Second, teach your . . ." Xiaojia Ge, et al., "Trajectories of Stressful Life Events and Depressive Symptoms During Adolescence," *Developmental Psychology*, Vol. 30, No. 4, 1994.

7. "Says Renee, eleven, . . ." Girls Inc.

8. "Other risk factors . . ." Lori Kowaleski-Jones and Frank Mott, research presented at Population Association of America meeting, May 1996.

9. "Punitive parenting styles . . ." Mark Sanford, et al., "Predicting the One-Year Course of Adolescent Major Depression," *Journal of the American Academy of Child and Adolescent Psychiatry*, Vol. 34, No. 12, December 1995.

10. "Children ages nine to . . ." *The Harvard Mental Health Letter*, "Mood disorders in childhood and adolescence, Part I," Vol. 10, No. 5, November 1993.

11. "Look for three clues . . ." Kathleen McCoy, Ph.D., *Understanding Your Teenager's Depression*, Perigree Books, 1994.

12. "The combination of . . ." *Brown University Child and Adolescent Behavior Letter*, "Keep Your Eye on Depression in Teenage Girls," Vol. 112, No. 1, 1996

13. "An estimated 5 percent . . ." Anxiety Disorders Association of America.

14. "While suicide rates . . ." ibid.

15. "Depressed children . . ." Jane Brody, "Suicide Myths Cloud Efforts to Save Children," *New York Times*, June 16, 1992.

16. "Girls, like boys . . ." ibid.

17. "A poll found . . ." Gallup Survey, "First National Survey on Teen Suicide," April 1991.

18. "Treatment of children . . ." Fishman.

Chapter 15: Violence and Personal Safety

1. "Your daughter should . . ." Barbara Mackoff, M.D., *Growing a Girl*, Dell Publishing, 1996.

2. "One poll found that . . ." Time/CNN poll, *Time*, May 10, 1999.

3. "According to one survey . . ." Gail Stennies, "Firearm storage practices and children in the home, United States, 1994," *Archives of Pediatric and Adolescent Medicine*, Vol. 153, No. 6, June 1999.

4. "Nationwide. 4.4 percent . . ." U.S. Centers for Disease Control and Prevention, Youth Risk Behavior Surveillance System, 1993.
5. "While boys are more . . ." M. Berton, S. Stoff, "Exposure to Violence and Post–Traumatic Stress Disorder in Urban Adolescents," *Adolescence*, Vol. 31, 1996.
6. "Children who witness . . ." Children's Express, 1993 conference.
7. "Witnessing violence at home . . ." Mark Singer, "Contributors to Violent Behavior among Elementary and Middle School Children," *Pediatrics*, Vol. 104, No. 4, Part 1, October 1999.
8. "More than half . . ." Ms. Foundation for Women.
9. "Girls who assault . . ." A. Cohall, et al., "Love Shouldn't Hurt," *Journal of the American Medical Women's Association*, special issue on adolescence, Vol. 54, No. 3, August 1999.
10. "Violence can also . . ." ibid.
11. "For this reason . . ." ibid.
12. "In one study, only 4 percent . . ." Lynn Harris, "The Hidden World of Dating Violence," *Parade*, September 22, 1996.
13. "About 70 percent of . . ." American Association of University Women, *Voices of a Generation: Teenage Girls on Sex, School and Self*, 1999.
14. "Harassment can start . . ." ibid.

Chapter 16: Education

1. "In the early 1990s . . ." American Association of University Women, *Shortchanging Girls, Shortchanging America*, 1994.
2. "While surveys tell us . . ." American Association of University Women, *Gender Gaps: Where Our Schools Still Fail Our Children*, October 1998.
3. "Consider these sobering . . ."
   • AAUW, 1999.
   • AAUW, 1999.
   • AAUW, 1999.
   • FIND/SVP and Grunwald Assoc., 1995.
   • Charles Piller, "The Gender Gap Goes High Tech," *Los Angeles Times*, August 25, 1998.
   • Maggie Ford, "The Silicon Ceiling," *Family PC*, March 1999.

4. "One study found that parents . . ." Sandi Kahn Shelton, "Girls and Money," *Working Mother*, September 1998.

5. "Women who take more . . ." Catherine Cartwright, "Daughters 2000," *Working Mother*, June 1999.

6. "All kids who intend . . ." Ms. Foundation, *Girls Seen and Heard*.

7. "It's no surprise . . ." Catherine Cartwright, "Daughters 2000," *Working Mother*, June 1998.

8. "If your daughter does . . ." Helen S. Farmer, "Why Some Women Persisted in Science Careers," presented at the American Psychological Association meeting, August 1994, Los Angeles.

9. "Teachers give boys . . ." AAUW, 1998.

10. "Girls tend to underestimate . . ." David A. Cole, "Children's Over- and Underestimation of Academic Competence," *Child Development*, Vol. 70, No. 2, March/April 1999.

11. "Studies show that children's . . ." Adele E. Gottfried, et al., "Role of Parental Motivation Practices in Children's Academic Intrinsic Motivation and Achievement," *Journal of Educational Psychology*, Vol. 86, No.1, March 1994.

12. "Concentrate on praising . . ." Claudia M. Mueller and Carol S. Dweck, "Praise for Intelligence Can Undermine Children's Motivation and Performance," *Journal of Personality and Social Psychology*, Vol. 75, No. 1, 1998.

13. "As children get older . . ." Child Trends, Inc., "Running in place: How American Families Are Faring in a Changing Economy and an Individualistic Society," 1994.

14. "This often leads . . ." Charlotte Milholland, *The Girl Pages*, Hyperion, 1998, section written by Whitney Ransome and Meg Moulton, of the National Coalition of Girls' Schools.

15. "There is good data . . ." Susan Estrich, "Separate is Better," *New York Times*, May 22, 1994.

16. "There is no good . . ." AAUW, 1998.

17. "Do you ever wonder . . ." Anne Chapman, "A Great Balancing Act," National Association of Independent Schools, 1997.

18. "As experts from . . ." *Girls Seen and Heard*.

19. "Spending too much . . ." Richard T. Cooper, Tini Tran, "Jobs Outside High School Can Be Costly, Report Finds," *Los Angeles Times*, November 6, 1998.

Chapter 17: Smoking

1. "When I started . . ." Shari Roan, "Struggle to Quit," *Los Angeles Times*, February 14, 2000.
2. "About 40 percent of all white . . ." U.S. Centers for Disease Control and Prevention, "Youth Risk Behavior Surveillance," Vol. 45, No. 55–4, September 27, 1996.
3. "Smoking is so likely . . ." Marlene Cimons, "FDA Chief Calls Nicotine Addiction a 'Pediatric Disease,' " *Los Angeles Times*, March, 9, 1995
4. "However, if you can . . ." Drug Strategies, "Keeping Score: Women and Drugs: Looking at the Federal Drug Control Budget," 1998.
5. "Your daughter needs . . ." ibid.
6. "About half of . . ." Elizabeth Gilpin and John Pierce, "How Long Will Today's New Adolescent Smoker Be Addicted to Cigarettes?" *American Journal of Public Health*, Vol. 86, No. 2, February 1996.
7. "Women who start . . ." *University of Connecticut Health and Science*, Vol. 4, No. 3, Spring 1999.
8. "Lung cancer rates . . ." U.S. Centers for Disease Control and Prevention and U.S. Department of Health and Human Services, "Priorities for Women's Health," Spring 1993.
9. "Cigarette smoking is . . ." American Cancer Society, "Cancer Facts & Figures," 1998.
10. "Women smokers have . . ." National Cancer Institute office of cancer communications, April 23, 1997.
11. "Yet, only about . . ." University of Connecticut.
12. "Smoking even a few . . ." Diane R. Gold, et al., "Effects of cigarette smoking on lung function in adolescent boys and girls," *New England Journal of Medicine*, Vol. 335, No. 13, September 26, 1996.
13. "Smoking also seems . . ." John K. Wiencke, et al., "Early Age at Smoking Initiation and Tobacco Carcinogen DNA Damage in the Lung," *Journal of the National Cancer Institute*, Vol. 91, No. 7, April 1999.
14. "It may be that . . ." University of Indiana press release, October 8, 1991.
15. "While it's not . . ." University of Connecticut.
16. "Kids begin smoking . . ." Irwin Sarason, et al., "Adolescents' Reasons for Smoking," *Health Psychology*, Vol. 62, No. 5, May 1992.
17. "Kids may choose . . ." University of Indiana.

18. "A pivotal reason . . ." Sandra G. Boodman, "Smoking to Stay Slim?" *Washington Post,* December 2, 1998, on research by Robert Klesges.

19. "Likewise, girls who . . ." Keeping Score.

20. "Parents who are extremely . . ." Deborah A. Cohen, "Parenting Behaviors and the Onset of Smoking and Alcohol Use: A Longitudinal Study," *Pediatrics,* Vol. 94, No. 3, September 1994.

21. "Parents who get . . ." ibid.

22. "Even preschoolers . . ." Christine L. Williams, M.D., remarks made at the American Heart Association seventy-first annual meeting.

23. "There is even some . . ." Denise B. Kandel, et al., "Maternal Smoking During Pregnancy and Smoking by Adolescent Daughters," *American Journal of Public Health,* Vol. 84, No. 9, September 1994.

24. "Finally, smoking advertising . . ." John Pierce, et al., "Smoking Initiation by Adolescent Girls: An Association with Targeted Advertising," *Journal of the American Medical Association,* Vol. 271, No. 8, 1994.

25. "Encourage your daughter . . ." Baylor University press release on research by Larry Laufman, et al., January 30, 1995.

26. "This rapid, repeated . . ." National Institute on Drug Abuse Research Report Series, July 1998.

27. "Keep in mind . . ." Steven H. Kelder, et al., "Longitudinal Tracking of Adolescent Smoking, Physical Activity, and Food Choice Behaviors," *American Journal of Public Health,* Vol. 84, No. 7, July 1994.

28. "Moreover, some . . ." UCLA News release, "Treating Nicotine Addiction Crucial by Age Eighteen," May 1999, on research by Stephen Shoptaw, Ph.D.

Chapter 18: Substance Abuse

1. "In 1999, five . . ." Meki Cox, "Inhalant Abuse: The Silent Epidemic," Associated Press, February 28, 1999

2. "The second major . . ." University of Michigan Monitoring the Future Survey, 1998.

3. "Today after twenty years . . ." National Institute on Drug Abuse, "Preventing Drug Use Among Children and Adolescents, A Research-based Guide," NIH, March, 1997, NIH Pub. No. 97–4214.

4. "African-American and Latino . . ." Lisa Guerra, M.D., remarks made at the Pediatric Academic Societies meeting, May 3, 1999.

5. "Many won't use . . ." C. Bodinger-de Uriarte, G. Austin, "Substance

Abuse Among Adolescent Females," *Prevention Research Update No. 9,* Northwest Regional Educational Laboratory.

6. "Thus, it is imperative . . ." NIDA, "Preventing Drug Use."

7. "The vast majority . . ." American Academy of Pediatrics press release, "New Findings on Teens and Underage Drinking," September 30, 1998.

8. "About 26 percent of . . ." U.S. Department of Health and Human Services, "Healthy Kids."

9. "While teen boys . . ." Drug Strategies, "Keeping Score: Women and Drugs: Looking at the Federal Drug Control Budget," 1998.

10. "Early use of alcohol . . ." HHS, "Healthy Kids."

11. "In 1997, one in four . . ." Drug Strategies.

12. "In the past . . ." Center on Addiction and Substance Abuse at Columbia University, "Report on College Drinking," June 7, 1994.

13. "Kids also say . . ." American Academy of Pediatrics.

14. "Nearly half of all . . ." ibid.

15. "A recent survey . . ." ibid.

16. "Use of this drug . . ." University of Michigan.

17. "Half of all kids . . ." ibid.

18. "And, like other drugs . . ." Drug Strategies.

19. "As many as 12 percent . . ." University of Michigan.

20. "These include . . ." NIDA.

21. "Teens who watch . . ." Reuters, "U.S. Teenage Drinking Linked to Watching More TV," November 2, 1998.

22. "A study of fifty . . ." Adam O. Goldstein, M.D., et al., "Tobacco and Alcohol Use in G-rated Children's Animated Films," *Journal of the American Medical Association,* Vol. 281, No. 2, March 24, 1999.

23. "One survey of twenty-eight . . ." Center for Medical Education, American Medical Association Media Briefing, March 18, 1999.

24. "It portrayed alcohol . . ." Mary Sue Coleman, president of the University of Iowa, Iowa City, personal correspondence.

25. "Point out that . . ." "Talking with Kids About Tough Issues," Children Now, Kaiser Family Foundation, 1996.

26. "When your daughter . . ." NIDA.

27. "The more parents talk . . ." Partnership for a Drug-Free America, April 1999.

28. "One of the most . . ." University of Southern California Health Sci-

ences News, "Study Shows 'Just Say No' Is Not Enough to Keep Kids Off Drugs," May 19, 1994.

29. "Many either deny . . ." Hazelden Foundation survey, 1996.
30. "About 77,000 teens . . ." Substance Abuse and Mental Health Services Administration (SAMHSA).
31. "Point out how . . ." SAMHSA guidelines.

Chapter 19: A Safe Environment

1. "Major difference in . . ." National Research Council, "Pesticides in the diets of infants and children," National Academic Press, Washington, D.C., 1993.
2. "They place their . . ." National Research Council and the U.S. EPA Conference, "Preventable Causes of Cancer in Children: A Research Agenda," *Environmental Health Perspectives*, 1998.
3. "In 1995, more than . . ." Mothers & Others, *The Green Guide*, No. 56/57, July 1, 1998.
4. "Boy and girls are both . . ." John Peters, M.D., et al., "A study of twelve Southern California Communities with differing levels and types of air pollution," *American Journal of Respiratory and Critical Care Medicine*, Vol. 159. No. 3, March 1999.
5. "Long-term exposure . . ." Ira Tager, M.D, et al., "Air pollution and lung function growth: is it ozone?" *American Journal of Respiratory and Critical Care Medicine*, Vol. 160, No. 2, August 1999.
6. "As many as . . ." *Journal of the National Institute for Environmental Health, Environmental Health Perspectives*, "Carcinogen Risk Assessment Guidelines on Children," Vol. 107, No. 6.
7. "No child should . . ." Mothers & Others.
8. "But as many as 4 percent . . ." ibid.
9. "Children drink twice . . ." Physicians for Social Responsibility, "Children's Environmental Health 1995 Report Card."
10. "Most cities have . . ." The ZPG Reporter, "Children's Environmental Index," Vol. 27, No. 3, July 1995.
11. "Unintentional injuries are . . ." National Safe Kids Campaign, 1994.
12. "About 8,000 . . ." National Center for Health Statistics, 1991.
13. "The good news . . ." National Safe Kids Campaign.

14. "Children at age seven . . ." Mattel Foundation, "Helping Kids Grow," 1994.
15. "Be vigilant all . . ." National Safe Kids Campaign.
16. "Riding unrestrained greatly . . ." ibid.
17. "Teens generally . . ." Kathleen O. Ryan, "Driving Parents Crazy," *Los Angeles Times*, May 18, 1997.
18. "If at all possible . . ." ibid.

Chapter 20: Health Care

1. "Both children and . . ." Kaiser Family Foundation, "Hearing Their Voices: A Qualitative Research Study on HIV Testing and High-Risk Teens," June 1999.
2. "Pediatricians who treat . . ." American Academy of Pediatrics, Policy Statement, "Update on Contraception and Adolescents," November 1, 1999.
3. "The Academy of . . ." Paula J. Hillard, M.D., remarks made at the American College of Obstetricians and Gynecologists briefing on adolescent health, December 9, 1997.
4. "In general, 'teen . . . ' " Kaiser Family Foundation.
5. "Many women today . . ." Shari Roan, "Special Report: A Checkup on Women's Health," *Los Angeles Times*, May 3, 1999, on research by the Kaiser Family Foundation.
6. "Despite the . . ." Mark A. Schuster, M.D., et al., "Communication Between Adolescents and Physicians about Sexual Behavior and Risk Prevention," *Archives of Pediatric and Adolescent Medicine*, September 12, 1996.
7. "One survey found . . ." ibid.
8. "This is particularly . . ." Kaiser Family Foundation.
9. "Teens will resist . . ." ibid.
10. "Raquel, sixteen, described . . ." ibid.
11. "One survey found . . ." The Commonwealth Fund Survey on the Health of Adolescent Girls, November 1997.
12. "Many girls typically . . ." ibid.
13. "Around the time . . ." Children of Alcoholics Foundation, *Opening Pandora's Box*, 1998.
14. "This fifteen-year-old . . ." Kaiser Family Foundation.

15. "Consent: . . ." For a full discussion, see *Teenage Health Care*, By Gail B. Slap, M.D., and Martha M. Jablow, Pocket Books, 1996.
16. "One survey found . . ." The Commonwealth Fund.
17. "Failure to understand . . ." American Medical Association, "Culturally Competent Health Care for Adolescents," 1994.
18. "More than one-quarter . . ." The Commonwealth Fund.
19. "About one-third . . ." ibid.
20. "Annual medical exams . . ." American Medical Association web site, "Your Child's Development."

Permissions

The Commonwealth Fund, "Survey of the Health of Adolescent Girls," 1997.

The American Medical Assn., Mark A. Schuster, M.D., Ph.D., et al. "Communication Between Adolescents and Physicians About Sexual Behavior and Risk Prevention," *Archives of Pediatric and Adolescent Medicine*, Vol. 150, September, 1996.

The American Medical Assn., Thomas L. Young, M.D., and Rick Zimmerman, Ph.D., "Clueless: Parental Knowledge of Risk Behaviors of Middle School Students," *Archives of Pediatric and Adolescent Medicine*, Vol. 152, November 1998.

KidsPeace, the National Center for Kids Overcoming Crisis, 1995 KidsPeace National Preteen Survey.

The Kaiser Family Foundation and Children Now, "Talking With Kids About Tough Issues," 1999.

Los Angeles Times, Shari Roan, "Suffering in Silence," Jan. 10, 1995; Shari Roan "Who's to Blame for Teen Pregnancy," July 9–12, 1995.

Ortho Dermatological.

Center for Media Literacy, Los Angeles, CA., "Parenting in a TV Age Resource Kit," 1991.

American Public Health Assn., Simone A. French, Ph.D., et al., "Frequent Dieting among Adolescents: Psychosocial and Health Behavior Correlates," May 1995, Vol. 85, No. 5. Nicole Evans, M.S., et al., "Adolescents' Perceptions of Their Peers Health Norms," August 1995, Vol. 85, No. 8. Copyright 1995 by the American Public Health Assn.

American College of Sports Medicine, "The Female Athlete Trial Position Stand Paper;" "Current Comment from the American College of Sports Medicine: Prevention of Sports Injuries of Children and Adolescents," August 1993; "Physical Activity, Genetic and Nutritional Considerations in Childhood Weight Management," July 1996.

The American Dietetic Association, "Child Nutrition and Health Campaign," copyright 1996. Used with permission.

International Life Sciences Institute, "Improving Children's Health Through Physical Activity: A New Opportunity," July 1997. Copyright 1997 International Life Sciences Institute.

American Council on Exercise, "Coax Your Kids Off the Couch and Onto a fun Fitness Routine," August 1997.

Sporting Goods Manufacturers' Association, "Tracking the Fitness Movement." Courtesy of the Dairy Management. Inc. TM/National Dairy Council, "National Teen Nutrition Research—Final Report, June 1996.

Frances M. Berg, *Children and Teens Afraid to Eat,* 2000 (revised edition), Healthy Weight Network.

Reprinted with permission from the Society for Nutritional Education, "Early Manifestations of Eating Disorders in Adolescents," Lucy B. Adams and Mary-Ann B. Shafer, M.D., *Journal of Nutrition Education,* Vol. 20, No. 6, 307–313, 1988.

"A Developmental Strategy to Prevent Lifelong Damage," David A. Hamburg, copyright 1995 Carnegie Corporation of New York. Reprinted with permission.

Courtesy of the City of Napa, CA, Police Department.

Girls Inc. Girls Incorporated is a national nonprofit organization responding to the needs of girls and their communities through programs, research, and advocacy designed to build girls' skills and self-confidence.

American Association of University Women Education Foundation, Washington, D.C., "Gender Gaps," and "Voices for a New Generation."

Walker Books, "The Repetitive Strain Injury Recovery Book," Deborah Quilter, 1998.

Copyright Mothers & Others for a Livable Planet.

Alvin Goldfarb; M.D., Professor of Obstetrics and Gynecology, Jefferson Medical College, Philadelphia, PA.

The National Council for Research on Women, "The Girls Report: What We Know and Need to Know About Growing Up Female," 1998.

From *See Jane Win* by Sylvia Rimm. Copyright (c) 1999 by Sylvia Rimm. Reprinted by permission of Crown Publishers, a division of Random House, Inc.

Index